Student Workbook to Accompany

Nadine Forbes, MS
Research Associate
Johns Hopkins University

Anatomy & Physiology
for Health Professions
An Interactive Journey

Bruce J. Colbert
Director of Allied Health
University of Pittsburgh at Johnstown

Jeff Ankney
Director of Clinical Education
University of Pittsburgh at Johnstown

Karen T. Lee
Associate Professor of Biology
University of Pittsburgh at Johnstown

PEARSON

Prentice
Hall

Upper Saddle River, New Jersey 07458

Pearson Prentice Hall™ is a trademark of Pearson Education, Inc.
Pearson® is a registered trademark of Pearson plc
Prentice Hall® is a registered trademark of Pearson Education, Inc.

Pearson Education LTD., *London*
Pearson Education Australia PTY, Limited, *Sydney*
Pearson Education Singapore, Pte. Ltd
Pearson Education North Asia Ltd, *Hong Kong*
Pearson Education, Canada, Ltd, *Toronto*
Pearson Educación de Mexico, S.A. de C.V.
Pearson Education—Japan, *Tokyo*
Pearson Education Malaysia, Pte. Ltd
Pearson Education, Inc. Upper Saddle River, New Jersey

ISBN 0-13-188976-1

CONTENTS

PREFACE

This workbook is designed to accompany the textbook *Anatomy and Physiology for Health Professions*. Many of its features will allow you to work at your own pace, helping you to evaluate your progress throughout the course. Answers are provided in an answer key at the end of the book. This workbook features a number of different ways to assess your progress as you journey through the text. Types of questions include:

Matching—In this section, there are three exercises per chapter in which you are asked to match chapter terminology and concepts with appropriate definitions.

Multiple Choice and Fill in the Blank—These sections provide an assessment to help test your knowledge of the chapter material

Short Answer—This section helps you to think critically and apply the chapter knowledge.

Labeling—In some chapters, you are asked to identify structures and label and/or color a blank image with the appropriate structures. These diagrams correspond to those found in the textbook.

We hope this workbook helps make your journey through anatomy and physiology an enjoyable one.

REVIEWERS

We would like to thank the following reviewers:

Eva Oltman, M.Ed.
Division Chair, Allied Health and Nursing
Jefferson Community and Technical College
Louisville, Kentucky

Sara K. Tallarovic, Ph.D.
Assistant Professor, Biology
University of the Incarnate Word
San Antonio, Texas

ANATOMY AND PHYSIOLOGY: LEARNING THE LANGUAGE

MULTIPLE CHOICE

1. Study of structure:
   a. Pathology
   b. Anatomy
   c. Physiology
   d. Cytology

2. Study of tissue structure and function:
   a. Cytology
   b. Dermatology
   c. Histology
   d. Anatomy

3. Study of function:
   a. Physiology
   b. Anatomy
   c. Pathology
   d. Cytology

4. The process of assessing the overall size and scarring pattern of the liver uses:
   a. Macroscopic anatomy
   b. Microscopic physiology
   c. Macroscopic cytology
   d. Microscopic histology

5. This system of measurement that is also called the International System:
   a. USCS
   b. British Imperial
   c. English
   d. Metric

6. The science and study of the causes of diseases and their modes of operation:
   a. Anatomy
   b. Hepatology
   c. Diseasology
   d. Pathology

7. A forecast of the probable course or outcome of a disease:
   a. Sign
   b. Prognosis
   c. Diagnosis
   d. Symptom

8. All chemical operations going on within the body:
   a. Metabolism
   b. Homeostasis
   c. Syndrome
   d. Pathology

9. Which system of measurement is used in places like the United Kingdom, Australia, and Canada?
   a. British Imperial
   b. Metric
   c. USCS
   d. a and c

10. In the English system, which is based on the British Imperial system, volume is expressed in:
    a. Milliliters
    b. Kilograms
    c. Pints
    d. Cubic centimeters

11. The foundation of a word is its:
    a. Prefix
    b. Root
    c. Suffix
    d. Etiology

12. In the U.S. Customary System, distance is expressed in:
    a. Feet
    b. Kilograms
    c. Centimeters
    d. Liters

13. In the metric system, weight is measured in:
    a. Pounds
    b. Liters
    c. Ounces
    d. Kilograms

14. Any abnormality indicative of disease and objectively discoverable on examination of a patient:
    a. Syndrome
    b. Symptom
    c. Sign
    d. Septic

15. The determination or identification of the nature of a disease, injury, or congenital defect:
    a. Sign
    b. Syndrome

c. Prognosis
    d. Diagnosis

16. Any subjective phenomenon or departure from the normal function or structure or sensation experienced by the patient or client:
    a. Prognosis
    b. Diagnosis
    c. Symptom
    d. Etiology

17. When the structure and/or function of the human body is disabled by virus, bacteria, and tissue death, the study of this state is termed:
    a. Proctology
    b. Parasitology
    c. Pathology
    d. Psychology

18. In breast feeding, the harder and more frequently the infant suckles, the more milk is produced and secreted from the mammary glands and ducts. This phenomenon is called:
    a. Metabolism
    b. Anabolism
    c. Negative feedback
    d. Positive feedback

19. The medical term for *outer layer of skin*:
    a. Dermatitis
    b. Epidermis
    c. Hypodermis
    d. Paradermotomy

20. Blood pressure is measured in terms of:
    a. Cubic centimeters
    b. Millimeter of mercury
    c. Liters
    d. IbHg

21. In the term *hypoglycemia*, its prefix is:
    a. hypo
    b. glyc/o
    c. emia
    d. glycemia

22. If *enter/o* means intestine, what then is painful, inflamed intestine?
    a. Enterology
    b. Paraenterotomy
    c. Enteritis
    d. Anenteromenorrhea

23. If *phleb/o* means vein, what is *inflammation of the vein?*
    a. Phlebitis
    b. Microphlebosis
    c. Acrophleboplasty
    d. Phlebalgiosis

24. Which of the following is considered a vital sign?
    a. Cyanosis
    b. Hypoglycemia
    c. Pulse
    d. Nausea

25. A physician who specializes in hearing disorders:
    a. Audiology
    b. Audiologist
    c. Audiotomy
    d. Audiophobia

MATCHING EXERCISES

Set 1

_____ 1. Phag/o   a. Sugar

_____ 2. Leuk/o   b. Blood

_____ 3. Hepat/o   c. Vessel

_____ 4. Glyc/o   d. Joint

_____ 5. Erythr/o   e. Liver

_____ 6. Dermat/o   f. Red

_____ 7. Angi/o   g. Bone

_____ 8. Gastr/o   h. Swallow

_____ 9. Oste/o   i. Stomach

_____ 10. Arthr/o   j. Skin

                           k. Intestine

                           l. White

Set 2

_____ 1. Slow   a. Otomy

_____ 2. Pain   b. Hyper

_____ 3. Difficult   c. Algia

_____ 4. Cutting into   d. Peri

_____ 5. Within   e. Hypo

_____ 6. Surgical removal of   f. Tachy

_____ 7. Small   g. Penia

_____ 8. Above normal   h. An

_____ 9. Below normal   i. Brady

_____ 10. Decrease or lack of   j. Endo

                                   k. Ectomy

                                   l. Micro

                                   m. Dys

Set 3

a. Anabolism
b. Vasoconstriction
c. Vasodilation
d. Acronym
e. Symptom
f. Syndrome

g. Etiology
h. Narcosis
i. Catabolism
j. Suffix
k. Sign

l. Positive feedback
m. Negative feedback
n. Prefix
o. Root word
p. Diagnosis

_____ 1. The way in which the body maintains a healthy body temperature despite an external environment that is extremely hot.

_____ 2. When the body breaks down substances into smaller components usable as energy sources.

_____ 3. When the body uses raw material like amino acids to build certain structures as protein molecule chains.

_____ 4. In the medical term osteochondritis, *osteochondr/o*.

_____ 5. The way in which the body maintains a healthy body temperature despite an external environment that is extremely cold.

_____ 6. Client A feels tired and lethargic, her skin is flushed, and she has a rapid pulse. The attending healthcare professional believes she has water intoxication (hyponatremia), probably from the marathon run 2 days prior. In terms of the presented disorder/dysfunction, *the lack of electrolytes during the marathon* would be its:

_____ 7. Client A feels tired and lethargic, her skin is flushed, and she has a rapid pulse. The attending healthcare professional believes she has water intoxication (hyponatremia), probably from the marathon 2 days prior. In terms of the client's condition, being *tired and lethargic* represents her:

_____ 8. Client A feels tired and lethargic, her skin is flushed, and she has a rapid pulse. The attending healthcare professional believes she has water intoxication (hyponatremia), probably from the marathon run 2 days prior. In terms of the presented disorder/dysfunction, *hyponatremia* is the:

_____ 9. Client A feels tired and lethargic, her skin is flushed, and she has a rapid pulse. The attending healthcare professional believes she has water intoxication (hyponatremia), probably from the marathon run 2 days prior. In terms of her condition, the rapid pulse would be its:

_____ 10. The mechanism, also termed *vicious cycle*, by which the body continues the response or magnifies the response to a stimulus:

FILL IN THE BLANK

1. The medical abbreviation for *immediately*: _____

2. The medical abbreviation for *nothing by mouth*: _____

3. The adjustment made in the human body to maintain a stable internal environment by opposing the stimulus: _____

4. The system of measurement most widely used in medical professions: _____

5. Using the principles of medical terminology, what is *surgical repair of a vessel?* _____

6. Using the principles of medical terminology, what is the *study of the skin?* _____

7. Using the principles of medical terminology, what is *inflammation of the liver?* _____

8. Cholecyst/ means gallbladder. Using the principles of medical terminology, *the removal of the gallbladder* is termed: _____

9. The general term for the physiological process that maintains a stable internal environment: _____

10. The cause of or a reasonable explanation for the manifestation of a disease: _____

11. The process of disease identification: _____

12. The prediction of a disease's outcome: _____

13. Cytology and histology are examples of: _____ anatomy

14. Regulation of body temperature is controlled by this part of the brain: _____

15. Blood pressure, body temperature, and respiratory rate are examples of _____ signs.

SHORT ANSWER

1. Contrast the terms *sign* and *symptom*.

_____

_____

_____

_____

2. Explain the two subdivisions of metabolism.

_____

_____

_____

_____

3. What does the study of anatomy and physiology entail?

_____

_____

_____

_____

4. What countries use the mathematical system based on the British
   Imperial system?

_____

_____

_____

_____

5. How does the body maintain homeostasis in a very cold environment?

_____

_____

_____

_____

THE HUMAN BODY: READING THE MAP

Chapter 2

MULTIPLE CHOICE

1. What structure separates the thoracic cavity from the abdominopelvic cavity?
   a. The navel
   b. The diaphragm
   c. The nipple
   d. The liver

2. A slice through the human body that parallels the long axis and extends from front to back, dividing the body into left and right sections, is called the:
   a. Frontal plane
   b. Median plane
   c. Horizontal plane
   d. Mid-transverse plane

3. Which is *not* part of the dorsal cavity?
   a. The oral cavity
   b. The spinal vertebrae
   c. The cranium
   d. All of the above

4. The appendix is found in which abdominal quadrant?
   a. Hypogastric
   b. Left inguinal
   c. Right lower
   d. Left lower

5. What is the correct term for the area anterior to the elbow, marked by the flex of the elbow, superficial veins, and a slight depression?
   a. Antecubital
   b. Anteradial
   c. Antebrachial
   d. Axillary

6. In anatomical position, how is the body positioned?
   a. Sitting with back straight, chest out, feet flat on the floor, and palms in neutral position
   b. Body erect, face and feet pointing forward
   c. Palms facing anteriorly, arms at the side
   d. b and c

7. Which plane divides the body and its parts into superior and inferior portions?
   a. Sagittal
   b. Midsagittal
   c. Cranial
   d. Transverse

8. Nearest to the point of origin:
   a. Distal
   b. Anterior
   c. Proximal
   d. Superior

9. The axillary region can be used to take temperature. Where is it?
   a. Armpit
   b. Ear
   c. Rectum
   d. Belly button

10. Towards the head:
    a. Superior
    b. Dorsal
    c. Inferior
    d. Distal

11. In reference to the antebrachium, where is the hand?
    a. Superior
    b. Distal
    c. Deep
    d. Proximal

12. Near the surface:
    a. Lateral
    b. Dorsal
    c. Ventral
    d. Superficial

13. Where are the kidneys?
    a. Right and left upper quadrant
    b. Right and left lower quadrants
    c. Pelvic cavity
    d. Hypogastric region

14. In reference to the nose, where is the mouth?
    a. Superior
    b. Lateral
    c. Medial
    d. Inferior

15. In reference to the skull, where is the brain?
    a. Superficial
    b. Deep
    c. Anterior
    d. Posterior

16. Brown fat can accumulate in various parts of the body, including behind the knees. What is the clinical name of this area?
    a. Peroneal region
    b. Plantar region
    c. Patellar region
    d. Popliteal region

17. What is the back of the head area called?
    a. Orbital region
    b. Buccal region
    c. Cervical region
    d. Occipital region

18. The dorsal cavity consists of which two cavities?
    a. Right and left pleural
    b. Right and left cerebral hemispheres
    c. Cranial and spinal
    d. Thoracic and pelvic

19. What is another term for *ventral?*
    a. Anterior
    b. Dorsal
    c. Posterior
    d. Cephalic

20. What is another term for *posterior?*
    a. Ventral
    b. Anterior
    c. Dorsal
    d. Caudal

21. The majority of the stomach is in what quadrant of the abdomen?
    a. Umbilical
    b. Left upper
    c. Right hypochondriac
    d. Lower thoracic

22. In reference to the shoulders, where is the head?
    a. Deep
    b. Proximal
    c. Superior
    d. Caudal

23. What structures are contained in the pleural cavities?
    a. Lungs
    b. Trachea
    c. Esophagus
    d. All of the above

24. The thoracic cavity contains the following organs:
    a. Lungs, heart, and stomach
    b. Brain, spinal cord, and eyes
    c. Heart, lungs, and esophagus
    d. Stomach, spleen, and lungs

25. The mediastinum is a subdivision of which cavity?
    a. Umbilical
    b. Epigastric
    c. Pleural
    d. Thoracic

MATCHING EXERCISES

Set 1

_____ 1. Prone   a. Toward the surface

_____ 2. Superior   b. Face up

_____ 3. Lateral   c. Caudal

_____ 4. Superficial   d. To the front

_____ 5. Proximal   e. Away from the point of origin

_____ 6. Distal   f. Away from the body's surface

_____ 7. Deep   g. Away from midline

_____ 8. Medial   h. Face down

_____ 9. Inferior   i. Toward the point of origin

_____ 10. Supine   j. Cephalic

                               k. To the back

                               l. Toward midline

Set 2

_____ 1. Cranial   a. Lungs, heart, and esophagus cavity (be specific)

_____ 2. Mediastinum   b. Spleen region

_____ 3. Abdominal   c. Urinary bladder cavity (be specific)

_____ 4. Thoracic   d. Pancreas quadrant

_____ 5. Dorsal   e. Brain cavity (be specific)

_____ 6. Pelvic   f. Lungs cavity (be specific)

_____ 7. Umbilical   g. Brain and spinal cord

_____ 8. Ventral   h. Liver cavity

_____ 9. Left hypochondriac   i. Lungs, liver, and uterus

_____ 10. Pleural   j. Between the lumbar regions

                               k. Between inguinal regions

                               l. Heart and esophagus cavity

Set 3

_____ 1. Fingers	a. Femoral
_____ 2. Forearm	b. Pedal
_____ 3. Foot	c. Sternal
_____ 4. Breastbone	d. Antebrachium
_____ 5. Neck	e. Orbital
_____ 6. Wrist	f. Digital
_____ 7. Thigh	g. Cervical
_____ 8. Lower back	h. Axillary
_____ 9. Eye area	i. Lumbar
_____ 10. Mouth	j. Carpal
	k. Oral

FILL IN THE BLANK

1. The opposite of ventral is _____.

2. The common name for the buccal region is the _____.

3. The _____ test actually assesses for appendicitis by applying resistant force to a raised right leg.

4. In the thorax, the only cavities that are paired are called the _____ cavities.

5. The plane that divides the body into anterior and posterior sections is called the _____ plane.

6. The plane that divides the body into superior and inferior sections is called the _____ plane.

7. The reproductive organs are located in a specific cavity called the _____ cavity.

8. Above the right inguinal region and below the right hypochondriac region is the _____ region.

9. Below the umbilical region is a region known as the _____ region.

10. The inguinal region is also called the _____ region.

11. When a person is laying face downward, that is said to be _____.

12. Medial to both the right and left hypochondriac regions is the _____ region.

13. In reference to the antebrachium, the brachium is

    _____.

14. In reference to the pleural cavities, the mediastinum is

    _____.

15. If the uterus is the point of origin and the vagina extends away from it, in clinical terms, the vagina is _____ to the uterus.

SHORT ANSWER

1. Describe the clinical divisions or quadrants of the abdominal region.

   _____

   _____

   _____

   _____

2. Give three examples in which the supine position is advantageous.

   _____

   _____

   _____

   _____

3. Using anatomical terms, direct an anatomist to the calf muscles from the patella.

   _____

   _____

   _____

   _____

4. Explain in clinical and directional terms structures of the lower extremity from the hips to the toes.

   _____

   _____

   _____

   _____

5. Describe the coronal plane.

   _____

   _____

   _____

   _____

LABELING ACTIVITY

Shade each cavity with a contrasting color and list a major structure or organ contained in this cavity beneath the corresponding label using Figure 2–7 on page 31 from your textbook as a guide.

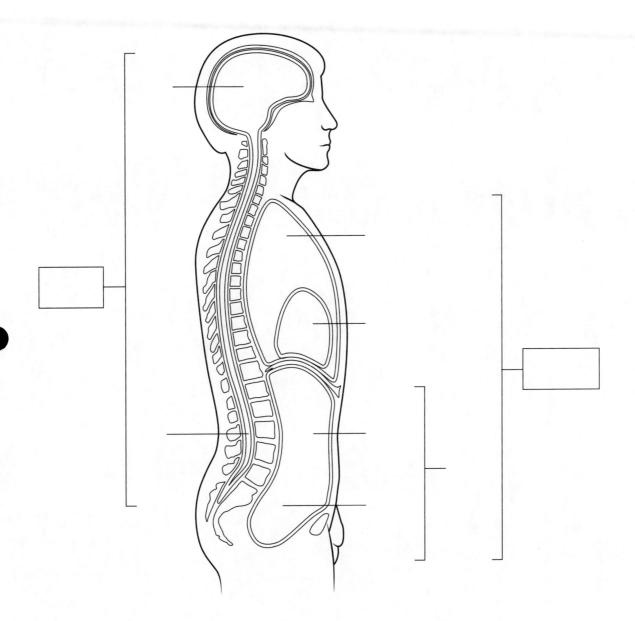

THE CELLS: THE RAW MATERIALS AND BUILDING BLOCKS

MULTIPLE CHOICE

1. The diffusion of water across a membrane is called:
   a. Diffusion
   b. Osmosis
   c. Phagocytosis
   d. Exocytosis

2. Where is DNA synthesized?
   a. Endoplasmic reticulum
   b. Lysosomes
   c. Golgi apparatus
   d. Nucleus

3. Which mechanism uses ATP?
   a. Exocytosis
   b. Pinocytosis
   c. Endocytosis
   d. All of the above

4. The microorganism that causes herpes is a:
   a. Bacterium
   b. Protozoan
   c. Virus
   d. Fungus

5. A sperm cell, if not mutated, propels itself with a single hairlike structure. This type of structure is called:
   a. Flagellum
   b. Cilium
   c. Tinea cordae
   d. Cordae equina

6. Containers A and B are separated by a semipermeable membrane. The solute concentration is 6mg/ml in container A and 2 mg/ml in container B. In what direction will *osmosis* take place?
   a. B to A
   b. No movement can take place
   c. A to B
   d. From A to B first and then from B to A for stability

7. What process occurs across the walls of small blood vessels, pushing both water and dissolved nutrients into the tissues of the body?
   a. Osmosis
   b. Diffusion
   c. Filtration
   d. Hemolysis

8. In what part of the nucleus are instructions for protein synthesis stored?
   a. RNA
   b. DNA
   c. Cilia
   d. Lysosome

9. When a membrane allows certain substances in and out, the membrane is said to be:
   a. Semipermeable
   b. Selectively permeable
   c. Impermeable
   d. a and b

10. What must every cell have in order to maintain its integrity and to survive?
    a. Nucleus
    b. Cilia
    c. Cell membrane
    d. Capsid

11. The inner membrane of the trachea moves phlegm upwards in a wavelike motion with its microscopic hairlike projections. These types of structures are called
    a. Flagella
    b. Cilia
    c. Endoplasmic reticula
    d. Receptors

12. The type of cellular transport that is moving substances against the concentration gradient:
    a. Diffusion
    b. Filtration
    c. Active pump
    d. Osmosis

13. Glucose needs to be ushered into the cells using:
    a. Facilitated diffusion
    b. Phagocytosis
    c. Pinocytosis
    d. Exocytosis

14. How can viruses nourish themselves?
    a. Being so unique, this microscopic organism has a mouthlike opening that pulls in debris and cells floating in the blood or interstitial fluid
    b. They must enter another cell and use that cell's parts for energy and growth material
    c. As long as exposed to light, they need not nourish
    d. Through the absorption of methane outside cellular sources

15. Which of the following is a type of transport through a cell membrane with or along the concentration gradient?
    a. Active transport pumps
    b. Diffusion
    c. Phagocytosis
    d. Exocytosis

16. The microorganism that causes athlete's foot is a:
    a. Bacterium
    b. Virus
    c. Fungus
    d. Protozoa

17. Postural muscles, such as muscles of the neck, are in constant need of energy. Therefore, these muscle cells contain and maintain higher quantities of what type of organelles than do cells not requiring high-energy stores?
    a. Mitochondria
    b. Nucleus
    c. Ribosomes
    d. Endoplasmic reticulum

18. What are the three main parts of a cell?
    a. Dendrite, axon, and soma
    b. Plasma membrane, cytoplasm, and nucleus
    c. Prophase, anaphase, and metaphase
    d. Cutaneous, serous, and mucous

19. A pathogen is:
    a. An organism that produces diseases
    b. A host for viruses
    c. A cellular receptor
    d. An internal method of transport

20. What is the function of the mycelia on fungi?
    a. Reproduction
    b. Absorb nutrients
    c. Cell division
    d. Movement

21. There are two classes of tumors. The life-threatening tumor is called:
    a. Malignant
    b. Sigma
    c. Bacteria
    d. Benign

22. When cardiac pressure forces plasma and various dissolved materials through the kidney membrane, this is an example of:
    a. Diffusion
    b. Facilitated diffusion
    c. Filtration
    d. Reno-exocytosis

23. An activated canister of tear gas is thrown into a room. Soon the gas has spread wall to wall and floor to ceiling. This movement of the gas is an example of:
   a. Diffusion
   b. Endocytosis
   c. Osmosis
   d. Pinocytosis

24. When a cancerous tumor breaks off and travels to other parts of the body, it is said to be:
   a. Thrombosized
   b. Embolized
   c. Metastasized
   d. Dormant

25. Candidiasis is common in some people suffering from AIDS. Candidiasis is a result of what type of infection?
   a. Protozoan
   b. Fungal
   c. Viral
   d. Bacterial

MATCHING EXERCISES

Set 1

_____ 1. Passive

_____ 2. Active

_____ 3. Diffusion

_____ 4. Filtration

_____ 5. Pinocytosis

_____ 6. Exocytosis

_____ 7. Endocytosis

_____ 8. Phagocytosis

_____ 9. Active transport pumps

_____ 10. Osmosis

a. Pressure is applied to force water and dissolved material across a membrane

b. Intake of liquid and food by cells by engulfing

c. Movement of substances from higher concentration to lower concentration

d. General term for a type of transport that requires energy

e. Movement of water from areas of low concentration of solute to areas that have high concentration of solute

f. How a cell transports things out of itself using a vesicle

g. General term for a type of transport that requires no energy

h. "Pushing" more into the cell using ATP as energy

i. Specifically, the intake of liquid by cells by engulfing

j. Specifically, the intake of solid particles by cells by engulfing

Set 2

_____ 1. Cell membrane

_____ 2. Nucleolus

_____ 3. Ribosome

_____ 4. Lysosome

_____ 5. Mitochondria

_____ 6. Endoplasmic reticulum

_____ 7. Golgi apparatus

_____ 8. Centrioles

_____ 9. Chromatin

_____ 10. Cytoplasm

a. A series of transport channels in the cell, having two distinct forms

b. Where RNA is synthesized

c. Produces ATP

d. Containing powerful enzymes

e. Contains DNA

f. Gel-like substance in which the cellular organelles float

g. Plays a critical role in cell division

h. Attaches to rough ER and produces protein

i. Surrounds the cells and allows certain substances in and other substances out

j. Packaging plant of a cell

Set 3

_____ 1. Bacteria

_____ 2. Malaria

_____ 3. Thrush

_____ 4. Virus

_____ 5. Pathogenic

_____ 6. Capsid

_____ 7. Streptococci

_____ 8. Shingles

_____ 9. Fungus

_____ 10. Protozoa

a. Microorganism that contributes to the normal flora of the body; can be pathogenic or nonpathogenic

b. The coat that surrounds the genetic material of a virus

c. Reoccurrence of chicken pox

d. An adjective used when an organism is said to produce diseases

e. Microorganism that cannot reproduce or eat by itself; needs a host

f. A disease caused by a protozoa living inside mosquitoes

g. General term for one-celled, animal-like organisms responsible for many tropical diseases transmitted through consumption of unclean water

h. Plantlike organism that can be either one-celled or multicelled

i. A disease of the mouth caused by a fungal infection

j. A disease of the throat caused by bacterial infection

FILL IN THE BLANK

1. The type of transport demonstrated by oxygen being transported from the lungs to the blood is _____.

2. When a cell surrounds a solid particle forming a vesicle and pulls it into the cells, this transport is called _____.

3. ATP stands for _____.

4. The situation in which more potassium is pulled into the cell despite being at a higher concentration inside the cell is called

_____.

5. The blueprint of the cell is contained in genetic material called

_____.

6. Of the two classes of tumors, the non-life-threatening one is a

_____ tumor.

7. The microorganism that is not killed by antibiotics is a

_____.

8. Certain bacteria in the intestine actually help synthesize vitamin

_____.

9. Fungi can spread through the release of _____.

10. The substance that is dissolved in water is referred to as the

_____.

11. The structural difference between ATP and ADP is the number of

_____ groups.

12. The type of microorganism that makes up the normal flora of the human body is the _____.

13. Most cells possess a nucleus. The exception is the

_____, which lacks a nucleus.

14. The smallest functional unit of the body is the _____.

15. A disease caused by a protozoa carried within the body of a mosquito is

_____.

SHORT ANSWER

1. What is the function of the cell membrane?

_____

_____

_____

_____

2. Identify places where protozoa live.

_____

_____

_____

_____

3. What are the common features of rough and smooth endoplasmic reticula?

_____

_____

_____

4. What is the difference between passive and active cellular membrane transport?

_____

_____

_____

5. Describe an example of filtration transport.

_____

_____

_____

_____

LABELING ACTIVITY

Label the parts of the cell using Figure 3–10 on page 56 of your textbook as a guide.

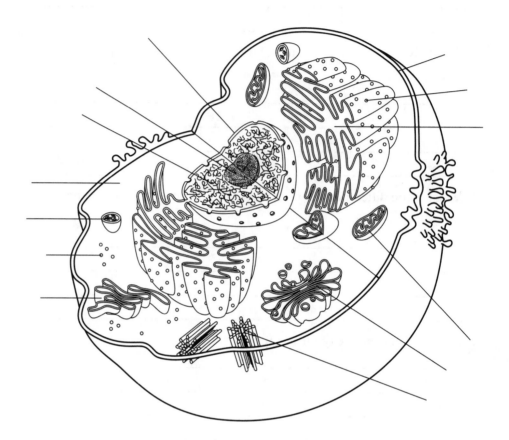

TISSUES AND SYSTEMS: THE INSIDE STORY

Chapter 4

MULTIPLE CHOICE

1. When an epithelial tissue is single-layered and made of flat, scale-like cells, what is it called?
   a. Simple scalular
   b. Unisqualous
   c. Simple squamous
   d. Monoplatino

2. The most common type of tissue in the body:
   a. Epithelial
   b. Connective
   c. Nervous
   d. Muscular

3. When an epithelial tissue is multiple-layered and made of cells that are taller than they are wide, what are they called?
   a. Stratified columnar
   b. Striated towercity
   c. Polypillarity
   d. Multirectangular

4. What is the clinical term for *fat*?
   a. Synovial tissue
   b. Parietal tissue
   c. Adipose tissue
   d. Sebaceous tissue

5. What is the function of the neuron?
   a. Conductor of information
   b. Producer of hormone
   c. Protection and support
   d. Storage of fat and protein

6. Which of the following epithelial tissues can be found in the outermost layer of skin?
   a. Polypillarity
   b. Striated scalular
   c. Stratified squamous
   d. Simple columnar

7. Which of the following epithelial tissues can be found lining the air sac of the lungs?
   a. Striated scalular
   b. Simple squamous
   c. Monorectangular
   d. Unipillarity

8. Blood and lymph are considered to be:
   a. Synovial tissue
   b. Connective tissue
   c. Serous tissue
   d. Mucous tissue

9. The membrane that lines cavities that open to the exterior, such as the mouth, reproductive, and respiratory tracts, is called:
   a. Mucous membrane
   b. Serous membrane
   c. Visceral membrane
   d. Cutaneous membrane

10. The visceral layer of a serous membrane:
   a. Lines the inside of the skull
   b. Wraps around the individual organs
   c. Holds neurons together
   d. Lines the body cavities

11. Which of the following statements is true about the internal structure of skeletal muscle cells?
   a. Multinucleated
   b. The only organelles present in the cytoplasm are mitochondria, giving the cell a striped appearance
   c. Has no nucleus
   d. Has no organelles

12. The parietal layer of serous membranes:
   a. Lines the body cavities
   b. Adheres to the brain and spinal cord
   c. Wraps around neuron to increase speed of impulse
   d. Lines the surface of the body

13. There is a membrane called *mesentery* that lines the abdominopelvic cavity and covers the organs. Taking this description into account, what type of membrane will this be considered?
   a. Cutaneous
   b. Mucous
   c. Serous
   d. Pseudocuboidal

14. Because it involves conscious effort and thought for movement, skeletal muscles are also called:
   a. Voluntary muscles
   b. Premeditated muscles
   c. Deliberate muscles
   d. Intentional muscles

15. Which of the following correctly describes the function of the mucus that mucous membranes produce and secrete?
    a. Nourishment
    b. Drying agent
    c. Digestive enzyme
    d. Lubrication

16. Each organ is a group of several different kinds of:
    a. Regions
    b. Systems
    c. Muscles
    d. Tissues

17. Because it does not require us to consciously think about its contractions, cardiac and visceral muscle tissues are considered what kind of muscles?
    a. Habitual
    b. Spontaneous
    c. Involuntary
    d. Instinctive

18. Which of the organs below are paired?
    a. Spleens
    b. Kidneys
    c. Livers
    d. Urinary bladders

19. What type of tissue is fat considered?
    a. Connective
    b. Epithelial
    c. Serous
    d. Cutaneous

20. Due to its microscopic appearance in comparison with the skeletal muscle, visceral muscle is also called:
    a. Little Swiss
    b. Smooth
    c. Rough
    d. Spongy

21. Which part of the neuron transmits impulses *toward* the cell body?
    a. Dendrite
    b. Soma
    c. Meninges
    d. Axon

22. The function of hormones:
    a. Regulate metabolic processes
    b. Regulate fluid balance
    c. Regulate rate of growth and reproduction
    d. All of the above

23. Where is visceral muscle found in the body?
    a. Digestive system
    b. Cardiovascular system
    c. Urinary system
    d. All of the above

24. The organ(s) below is/are considered vital organs:
    a. Gallbladder
    b. Appendix
    c. Brain
    d. All of the above

25. Which body system *stores* the mineral calcium?
    a. Circulatory
    b. Digestive
    c. Lymphatic
    d. Skeletal

MATCHING EXERCISES

Set 1

_____ 1. Nervous tissue

_____ 2. Muscle tissue

_____ 3. Connective tissue

_____ 4. Epithelial tissue

_____ 5. Striated

_____ 6. Stratified

_____ 7. Serous

_____ 8. Meninges

_____ 9. Cutaneous

_____ 10. Synovial

a. Specifically, the *membrane* that covers the spinal cord and brain

b. Tissue, the systemic job of which is to hold things together and provide structure

c. Appearance of skeletal muscles

d. Has the ability to shorten itself; provides movement by and in our bodies

e. Epithelial tissue of more than one layer of cells

f. Found in the space between bone joints and produces a slippery fluid

g. *Membrane* that covers both organs and cavities

h. Communication; rapid messenger of information

i. Commonly known as the skin

j. The *tissue* type that covers the body and its parts

Set 2

_____ 1. Lymphatic system

_____ 2. Endocrine system

_____ 3. Nervous system

_____ 4. Female reproductive system

_____ 5. Male reproductive system

_____ 6. Digestive system

_____ 7. Respiratory system

_____ 8. Integumentary system

_____ 9. Cardiovascular system

_____ 10. Muscular system

a. Supports and sustains structure; framework of body

b. Movement; controls the diameter of blood vessels

c. Surface protection from harmful environmental invaders

d. Produces ova and houses the growing fetus

e. Communication and control through the release of chemical substances

f. Produces red blood cells

g. Chemically and mechanically breaks down food for use by the body

h. Communication transmission of impulses

i. Transports water, oxygen, and nutrients to and away from the cells of the body

j. Produces sperm

k. Maintains proper fluid balance in the body; helps fight disease

l. Supplies fresh oxygen for the blood to absorb

Set 3

_____ 1. Both pancreas and testes

_____ 2. Both vas deferens and penis

_____ 3. Tonsils and lymph vessels

_____ 4. Heart and veins

_____ 5. Small intestine and gallbladder

_____ 6. Kidneys

_____ 7. Sweat and oil glands

_____ 8. Brain and spinal cord

_____ 9. Trachea and bronchus

_____ 10. Uterus and fallopian tubes

a. Belong to the system that produces sperm

b. Belong to the system that produces urine

c. Belong to the system that digests and eliminates food

d. Belong to the system that contains sensory and motor neurons

e. Belong to the system that produces hormones

f. Belong to the system that allows us to flex and extend bones at moveable joints

g. Belong to the system that covers and protects the body

h. Belong to the system that allows for the union of the sperm and ova

i. Belongs to the system that eliminates carbon dioxide from the body

j. Belong to the system that includes blood

k. Belong to the system that cleans up excess fluid and fights infections

FILL IN THE BLANK

1. Both visceral and parietal membranes are part of _____ membranes.

2. The organ with which cardiac muscle is associated is called the _____.

3. A neuron is one type of nerve cell; the other type of nerve cell is called _____.

4. The testes belong to the reproductive and the _____ systems.

5. The pancreas belongs to the endocrine and the _____ systems.

6. Hormones circulate through the _____ system.

7. Sight, hearing, touch, taste, and smell belong to the _____ system.

8. The skin has the ability to produce vitamin _____.

9. The part of the neuron called the _____ transmits impulses away from the cell body.

10. Pseudostratified _____ tissues line the lower part of the digestive tract.

11. The common feature of the lungs and kidneys is that both are _____, so if one is damaged, you will still survive.

12. When muscles are striped in appearance, they are said to be _____.

13. The membrane that lines joints produces a fluid that reduces friction called _____.

14. Tendons and ligaments are composed of dense _____ tissue.

15. The spleen belongs to the _____ system.

SHORT ANSWER

1. List and describe the four main types of tissues.

_____

_____

_____

_____

2. Differentiate the three main types of muscle tissue.

_____

_____

_____

_____

3. Describe the main components of nerve tissue.

_____

_____

_____

_____

4. Describe the functions of a serous membrane.

_____

_____

_____

_____

5. Compare the similarities of the endocrine and the nervous systems.

_____

_____

_____

_____

LABELING ACTIVITY

Color and label each type of tissue using Figure 4–1 on page 71 of your textbook as a guide.

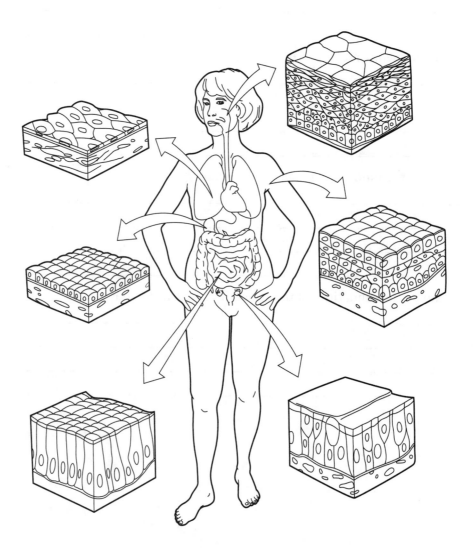

THE SKELETAL SYSTEM: THE FRAMEWORK

Chapter 5

MULTIPLE CHOICE

1. When a fracture breaks the skin:
   a. Simple fracture
   b. Closed fracture
   c. Compound fracture
   d. a and b

2. Please identify which of the choices below is a nutritional disorder.
   a. Gigantism
   b. Kyphosis
   c. Rickets
   d. Osteosarcoma

3. Osteomyelitis is an example of:
   a. An infection
   b. A congenital disorder
   c. A trauma
   d. A tumor

4. Which of the following allows your body to absorb ingested calcium from the digestive tract?
   a. Iron
   b. Vitamin B_{12}
   c. Vitamin D
   d. Phosphorus

5. Which of the following vices, according to your text, decreases bone mass?
   a. Caffeine: coffee or Mountain Dew
   b. Tobacco: cigarette smoking
   c. Bourbon: overindulgence in the spirits
   d. Chocolate: constantly feeding a Hershey's craving
   e. a and b
   f. a, b, c, d

6. What happens to ligaments and tendons when we age?
   a. Change from a bluish tint to an opaque yellow
   b. Degenerate, becoming more flexible and loose, leading to increased range of motion, increased sprains, and more propensity for dislocations
   c. Become less flexible, leading to decreased range of motion
   d. Slowly detach from their attachment bones

7. What is the function of osteoblasts?
   a. Tear down bone
   b. Build new bone
   c. Absorb calcium from the gut
   d. Stimulate calcium retention in the kidneys

8. Where are osteoprogenitor cells found?
   a. Periosteum
   b. Spleen
   c. Bone marrow
   d. Thymus

9. The primary component of the skeleton is:
   a. Synovial fluid
   b. Cartilage
   c. Bone
   d. Ligament

10. The phalanges and ulna are examples of what type of bone?
    a. Irregularly shaped
    b. Long
    c. Short
    d. Flat

11. The mandible and cervical vertebrae are examples of what type of bone?
    a. Irregularly shaped
    b. Long
    c. Short
    d. Flat

12. The parietal and scapulae bones are examples of what type of bone?
    a. Irregularly shaped
    b. Long
    c. Short
    d. Flat

13. The expanded ends of long bone are called:
    a. Epimysia
    b. Epicondyles
    c. Epiphysis
    d. Epiosteum

14. What substance is housed in the medullary cavity, yet absent in the trabeculae?
    a. Progenitor cells
    b. Yellow bone marrow
    c. Red bone marrow
    d. Digestive enzymes

15. What type of bony tissue makes up the adult diaphysis?
    a. Cancellous bone
    b. Spongy bone
    c. Cartilage
    d. Compact bone

16. Mature bone cells are clinically called:
    a. Osteocytes
    b. Osteoblasts
    c. Osteoprogenitor
    d. Osteoclasts

17. The formation of red blood cells:
    a. Hemopoiesis
    b. Hemoglobin
    c. Hematocytosis
    d. Erythrogenesis

18. Nodding the head in an aggressive gesture of "yes" is employing:
    a. adduction/abduction
    b. rotation
    c. flexion/extension
    d. supination/pronation

19. Connective tissue that attaches muscle to bone:
    a. Tendon
    b. Cartilage
    c. Ligament
    d. Fascia

20. Moving the joints of the ankle and foot so that the sole of one foot is facing away from the other:
    a. Pronation
    b. Eversion
    c. Hyper adduction
    d. Plantar flexion

21. Which of the following bones belongs to the axial skeleton?
    a. Clavicle
    b. Scapula
    c. Hyoid
    d. Tarsal

22. Which of the following bones belongs to the appendicular skeleton?
    a. Ribs
    b. Sternum
    c. Ilium
    d. Sacrum

23. The tip of the sternum is called the:
    a. Xyphoid
    b. Hyoid
    c. Condyloid
    d. Patella

24. The vertebral column has how many vertebrae in the midbuttocks region, neck region, lower back, and upper back region?
    a. 7, 12, 5, 5
    b. 3–4, 12, 5, 5
    c. 5, 7, 5, 12
    d. 1–4, 7, 12, 5

25. Besides depression and elevation, which of the following is also an action of the human mandible?
a. Protraction and retraction
b. Supination and pronation
c. Inversion and eversion
d. Flexion and extension
e. Rotation

MATCHING EXERCISES

Set 1

_____ 1. True ribs	a. Clavicle
_____ 2. Shoulder blade	b. Metatarsals
_____ 3. Upper arm bone	c. Scapula
_____ 4. Fingers and toes	d. Radius
_____ 5. Thigh bone	e. Femur
_____ 6. Lower leg bone	f. Vertebrocostal
_____ 7. Forearm bone	g. Fibula
_____ 8. Wrist bones	h. Tarsals
_____ 9. Ankle bones	i. Phalanges
_____ 10. Foot bones	j. Humerus
	k. Carpals
	l. Metacarpals
	m. Vertebrosternal

Set 2

_____ 1. Ellipsoidal

_____ 2. Synovial

_____ 3. Ball and socket

_____ 4. Gliding

_____ 5. Saddle

_____ 6. Pivot

_____ 7. Condyloid

_____ 8. Cartilaginous

_____ 9. Fibrous

_____ 10. Hinge

a. Neck and forearm; rotates

b. Found at the pubic symphysis and joining the ribs to the sternum

c. Hips and shoulder; multiple movement

d. Knees and elbow; allows for flexion and extension

e. Found on the cranium; sutures

f. Base of the thumb; multiple movement including opposition

g. Fluid in a joint cavity

h. Knuckles, oval-shaped bone ends; allows for adduction/abduction

i. Found between the carpals and between the tarsals

j. Found between wrist bones and the forearm bones; allows biaxial movement

Set 3

_____ 1. Diaphysis

_____ 2. Facet

_____ 3. Tubercle

_____ 4. Fossa

_____ 5. Meatus

_____ 6. Sinus

_____ 7. Crest

_____ 8. Head

_____ 9. Foramen

_____ 10. Spine

a. A tube or tunnellike passageway through a bone

b. A nontubular passageway through a bone for ligaments, nerves, and blood vessels

c. A small flattened area

d. The shaft of the bone

e. A knob-like projection

f. A sharp pointed projection

g. A hollow area; space within a bone

h. An articulating end of a bone that is rounded

i. A narrow ridge

j. Shallow depression

FILL IN THE BLANK

1. The medical condition called _____ is a degenerative disorder characterized by a decrease in bone density.

2. Cleft palate and club foot are examples of _____ disorders.

3. Secondary curvatures of the spine are found in the _____ and _____ vertebral regions.

4. According to your text, osteoclasts arise from _____.

5. If you move the joint of the ankles and foot so that you are "standing" on the balls of the foot, you have then _____ the foot.

6. When a joint is straightened or merely moved so that the angle between the individual bones has increased, the movement is termed _____.

7. The bone called the _____ is commonly known as the lower jaw.

8. During CPR chest compressions, the part called the _____ of the sternum takes the brunt of the compressive force.

9. Ribs 8, 9, and 10 can be clinically called _____, or commonly called false ribs.

10. Similar to the elbow joint, interphalangeal joints are _____ joints.

11. In the creation of the skeletal bones, when shaped cartilage is replaced by osseous tissue, this process is known as _____.

12. Where bursitis is inflammation of a bursa, inflammation of the joint is called _____.

13. The human skeleton has _____ bones.

14. Falling off his skateboard, Hugh suffered a _____ fracture due to the bones of his forearm being crushed to the point of splintering.

15. Specialized cells called _____ are needed to tear down bone.

SHORT ANSWER

1. What are four functions of the skeleton?

_____

_____

_____

_____

2. Compare and contrast the four types of bone.

_____

_____

_____

_____

3. What are the functions of the periosteum?

_____

_____

_____

_____

4. Discuss the difference between a ligament and a tendon.

_____

_____

_____

_____

5. Why are ribs 11 and 12 called floating ribs?

_____

_____

_____

_____

LABELING ACTIVITY

Label and color the parts of the bone indicated below using Figure 5–3 on page 101 from your textbook as a guide.

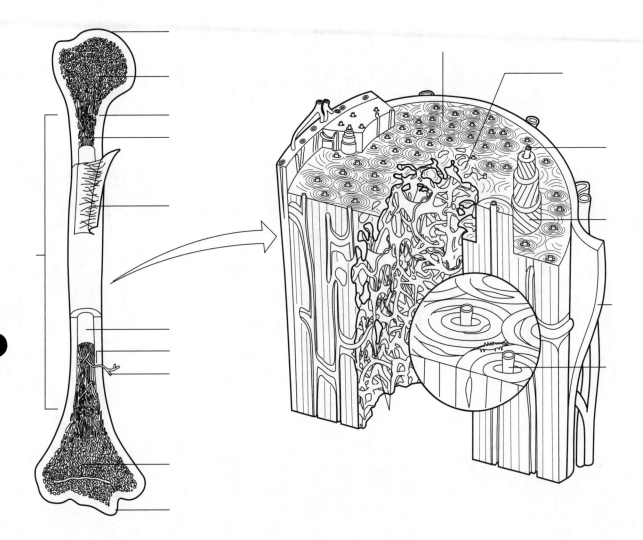

THE MUSCULAR SYSTEM: MOVEMENT FOR THE JOURNEY

Chapter
6

MULTIPLE CHOICE

1. Choose the correct structural arrangement from macro to micro in terms of size.
   a. Muscle cells, myofibrils, sarcomere, myofilament
   b. Myofibril, myofilament, muscle cell, sarcomere
   c. Myofilament, muscle cells, myofibrils, sarcomere
   d. Muscle cell, myofilament, sarcomere, myofibrils

2. Which of the following is a group of anterior thigh muscles?
   a. Hamstrings
   b. Quadriceps
   c. Peroneals
   d. Gluteals

3. Which of the following is a group of buttocks muscles?
   a. Psoas
   b. Gluteal
   c. Hamstrings
   d. Quadriceps

4. Which of the following is a muscle of the lower leg?
   a. Gastrocnemius
   b. Latissimus dorsi
   c. Deltoid
   d. Hamstring

5. Muscles that are used for duration or high endurance activity will:
   a. Look white due to the excess oxygen and fat stored for energy
   b. Look white due to the lack of blood supply
   c. Look dark due to the rich blood supply to carry needed oxygen
   d. Look dark due to chronic tears and scar tissue in the muscle fibers

6. Where are calcium ions stored in the muscle cells?
   a. End bulb
   b. Nucleus
   c. Myosin crossbridges
   d. Sarcoplasmic reticulum

7. Which of the following muscles is under voluntary control?
   a. Skeletal
   b. Cardiac
   c. Visceral
   d. Smooth

8. After death, when the body becomes stiff due to unreleased muscle contraction, the condition is referred to as:
   a. Rigor mortis
   b. Tetanus
   c. Myalgia
   d. Paralysis

9. When the diameter of a blood vessel increases:
   a. The pressure also increases
   b. It is termed vasoconstriction
   c. The pressure decreases
   d. b and c

10. An injury to a ligament:
    a. Strain
    b. Sprain
    c. Staine
    d. Stereophrane

11. Which of the following correctly describes an aponeurosis?
    a. A psychosis in which pain is felt in an area of a limb that has been amputated
    b. Inability to move the neck muscles
    c. A flat, broad, tendonlike sheath
    d. Necrosis (death) of the muscle cells

12. Why are migratory birds' breasts dark (as in the King Eider, Arctic Tern, and Blue Winged Teal) and nonmigratory birds' breasts white (as in the Turkey, Sandhill Crane, and Red Cardinal)?
    a. Migratory birds need speed to traverse far distances; dark meat is a clear attribute for speed
    b. Nonmigratory birds need endurance to traverse far distances; dark meat is a clear attribute for endurance
    c. Migratory birds need endurance to traverse far distances; dark meat is a clear attribute for endurance
    d. Nonmigratory birds need speed to traverse far distances; white meat is a clear attribute for endurance

13. What is/are energy source(s) used by muscle?
    a. Calcium
    b. Fat
    c. Glucose
    d. b and c

14. Which of the following is true about the sliding filament theory and consequently about muscle contraction?
    a. Crossbridges are formed between actin and myosin; myosin rotates, pulling the actin toward the center of the sarcomere

b. Crossbridges are formed between actin and the Z-lines; Z-lines rotate, and as a result, myosin shortens

c. Crossbridges are formed between actin and myosin; actin rotates, pulling myosin toward the Z-lines, shortening the sarcoplasmic reticulum

d. Sarcoplasmic reticulum releases phosphorous, resulting in crossbridges forming between myosin and the Z-lines; actin rotates, pulling toward the center of the sarcomere

15. Some sphincters are examples of:
   a. Skeletal muscle
   b. Smooth muscle
   c. Visceral muscle
   d. b and c

16. If the erector spinae muscles are the antagonist, which of the following will be a prime mover?
   a. Latissimus dorsi
   b. Trapezius
   c. Rectus abdominis
   d. a and b

17. One of the calf muscles, called the soleus, when contracted moves the heel of the foot (calcaneus) closer to the posterior leg. Given this information and your knowledge of the principles of origin and insertion, what is the muscle's origin?
   a. Calcaneus
   b. Anterior leg
   c. Posterior leg
   d. a and b

18. A group of muscles called the scalenes laterally flexes the neck. Given this information and your knowledge of the principles of origin and insertion, which of the following most likely is its insertion?
   a. Cervical vertebrae
   b. Shoulder
   c. Ribs
   d. Collarbone

19. Besides a physical separation of the thoracic cavity and the abdominal cavity, what purpose does the diaphragm serve?
   a. Flexes the trunk
   b. Extends the trunk
   c. Controls breathing
   d. All of the above

20. The diaphragm is what type of muscle?
   a. Smooth
   b. Cardiac
   c. Visceral
   d. Skeletal

21. The diaphragm is under what type of control?
    a. Voluntary
    b. Involuntary
    c. Both voluntary and involuntary
    d. Neither voluntary nor involuntary

22. A muscle called the deltoid pulls the arm away from the body, directly out away from the sides. This movement is referred to as:
    a. Rotation
    b. Abduction
    c. Adduction
    d. Lateral flexion

23. Which of the following muscles are striated?
    a. Sphincters
    b. Walls of blood vessels
    c. Muscles that move the upper arm
    d. Muscles of peristalsis

24. When the diameter of a blood vessel decreases:
    a. The pressure also decreases
    b. It is termed vasoconstriction
    c. The pressure increases
    d. b and c

25. Muscles that extend the forearm at the elbow most likely will have their bellies (bulging part) located in the:
    a. Anterior forearm
    b. Anterior arm
    c. Posterior forearm
    d. Posterior arm

MATCHING EXERCISES

Set 1

_____ 1. Latissimus dorsi a. Muscle encircling the mouth

_____ 2. Pectoralis major b. Muscle encircling the eyes

_____ 3. Rectus abdominis c. Muscle to the side of the jaw

_____ 4. Erector spinae d. Neck muscle

_____ 5. Orbicularis oculi e. Chest muscle

_____ 6. Masseter f. Vertical muscle from inferior margin of rib cage to the pubis

_____ 7. Orbicularis oris g. Lateral abdominal muscle

_____ 8. Mentalis h. Back muscle running from the vertebrae to the upper arm

_____ 9. Sternocleido-mastoid i. Vertical back muscle running from lower vertebrae to upper vertebrae

_____ 10. External obliques

j. Muscle of the mid chin

Set 2

_____ 1. Flexion
_____ 2. Rotation
_____ 3. Abduction
_____ 4. Extension
_____ 5. Adduction
_____ 6. Vasodilate
_____ 7. Vasoconstrict
_____ 8. Tetanus
_____ 9. Antagonist
_____ 10. Agonist

a. Prime mover

b. Lengthens upon movement or contraction of prime mover

c. Movement away from midline

d. Movement toward midline

e. Movement decreasing angle of the joint

f. Movement increasing the angle of the joint

g. Movement decreasing the diameter of the blood vessel

h. Movement increasing the diameter of the blood vessels

i. Movement around a center axis

j. Movement that creates rigid paralysis

Set 3

_____ 1. Myalgia
_____ 2. Hernia
_____ 3. Strain
_____ 4. Cramp
_____ 5. Sprain
_____ 6. Myasthenia gravis
_____ 7. Guillain-Barré syndrome
_____ 8. Botulism
_____ 9. Atrophy
_____ 10. Muscular dystrophy

a. Tear or injury in muscle and/or tendon

b. Involuntary, sudden, and violent contractions

c. Tears or breaks in a ligament

d. A PNS disorder resulting in flaccid paralysis

e. A disorder in which patients experience progressive yet gradual muscle weakness

f. Inherited muscle disease in which muscle fibers degenerate

g. A potentially deadly disease that causes paralysis and is a result of ingested bacteria

h. Tenderness and pain in muscle

i. A tear in a muscle wall through which an organ protrudes

j. Condition marked by rigid muscle spasm caused by a bacteria most likely entering the body via a puncture wound

k. The process of muscle wasting away; could be due to lack of nutrition, disease, or disuse

FILL IN THE BLANK

1. A structure called _____ allows for uniform contraction of the cardiac muscle.

2. The rhythmic internal movement of food products through the GI tract is termed _____.

3. The _____ muscle is the antagonist of the biceps brachii.

4. A muscle called the palmaris longus pulls the hand closer to the front of the forearm. This action at the wrist is known as _____.

5. In order to generate heat, the body _____, a biological reaction figuratively saying it is too cold.

6. In order to supply energy and heat, the body converts stored _____ into glucose.

7. The functional unit of the muscle is the _____.

8. Rigor mortis occurs when _____ cannot exit the sarcoplasmic reticulum.

9. Neurons secrete a neurotransmitter called _____, which sets the process of muscle contraction in motion.

10. Each functional unit of the muscle is separated from each other by _____.

11. Provided that the hamstrings are the prime movers, the _____ are the antagonists.

12. The group of muscles called the _____ assists the prime movers in a particular movement.

13. Smooth muscle is also called _____ muscle.

14. Cardiac muscle forms the walls of the _____.

15. A fibrous tissue attaching bone to bone is a _____.

SHORT ANSWER

1. Why does smooth muscle form scars rather than effectively healing itself?

_____

_____

_____

_____

2. Besides movement, what are two other very important functions of the muscular system?

_____

_____

_____

_____

3. Describe four places where smooth muscle can be found in the body.

_____

_____

_____

_____

4. What gives muscle its striped appearance?

_____

_____

_____

_____

5. List and describe three types of muscle tissue.

_____

_____

_____

_____

⬤ LABELING ACTIVITY

Label the muscles and color them for contrast using Figure 4–8 on page 81 of
your textbook as a guide.

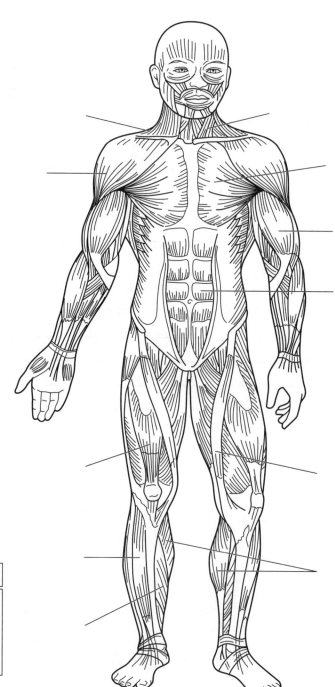

Organ	Primary Functions
Skeletal muscles (700)	Provide skeletal movement, control openings of digestive tract, produce heat, support skeletal position, protect soft tissues

THE INTEGUMENTARY SYSTEM: THE PROTECTIVE COVERING

MULTIPLE CHOICE

1. Hair is composed of a protein called:
   a. Hemoglobin
   b. Lanugo
   c. Lunago
   d. Keratin

2. The skin condition caused by the herpes simplex virus forming a visible lesion on the lip margins:
   a. Psoriasis
   b. Pustule
   c. Cold sore
   d. Acne

3. Usually observed in children, this contagious disease is caused by mites.
   a. Mumps
   b. Chicken pox
   c. Scabies
   d. Hives

4. "Jock itch" is caused by which of the following?
   a. Fungi
   b. Viruses
   c. Bacteria
   d. Protozoa

5. Some people of historic European descent have a pinkish tone to their skin because of
   a. Melanin
   b. Carotene
   c. Lack of melanocytes
   d. Surface vascularizaton

6. Which of the following correctly describes an abrasion?
   a. Raised skin, pimples with a defined border
   b. Open, crater-like sore where tissue death is evident
   c. Scratched off skin
   d. Bruise

7. Acne develops when:
   a. Glucose in consumed sweets solidifies in the sebaceous glands
   b. There is an overproduction of sebum and an inflammation of the oil glands
   c. Blockage of the sweat glands with dirt and environmental grime
   d. Sweat becomes too sweet, and viruses are attracted and accumulate at the pore opening

8. In a cold environment, blood vessels of the skin:
   a. Vasoconstrict, channeling blood from the periphery to the core in order to collect more blood cells and fibroblasts
   b. Vasodilate, accepting more blood from the body's core in order to be warmed by solar energy
   c. Vasoconstrict, channeling blood from the periphery toward the body's core where heat is
   d. Vasodilate, accepting blood from the body's core in order to dissipate heat at the skin's surface

9. To which of the following structures do the arrector pili muscles attach?
   a. Hair follicle
   b. Stratum corneum
   c. Elastin
   d. Subcutaneous fascia

10. Based on the information given in Chapter 7, in order for effective body cooling to occur:
    a. Water from sweat glands is excreted onto the skin, then is evaporated off, dispelling heat from the surface
    b. Water from sweat glands is excreted onto the skin, then as soon as it is felt, needs to be wiped off, carrying heat with the towel or cloth used
    c. Urination needs to cease, and excessive water consumption must be temporarily stopped
    d. Sweat needs to be at the body's core temperature, and nitrogenous wastes must be absent in the sweat excretion

11. What determines the texture of hair?
    a. Shaft shape: flat shafts produce curly hair, and round shafts produce straight hair
    b. Follicle shape: vertical follicles produce straight hair, and angular follicles produce curly hair
    c. Pigmentation: higher concentrations of pigmentation produce curly hair
    d. Heat and humidity: people exposed to cold will grow straight hair and people exposed to heat will not
    e. Diet: people consuming food high in folic acid will produce straight hair

12. What determines the color of hair?
    a. Carotene
    b. Melanin
    c. Keratin
    d. Bilirubin

13. Why should you not squeeze blackheads?
    a. May create a pit
    b. Substance in the pores and glands is highly contagious
    c. May force the infection back into the sudoriferous pore
    d. All of the above

14. What is/are the danger(s) of washing the face too often with non-pH-balanced soap?
    a. Loss of pigmentation
    b. Decrease blood supply
    c. Loss of nerve sensation
    d. Loss of antibacterial barrier
    e. All of the above

15. Shaving or frequent trimming will:
    a. Cause hair to grow faster
    b. Cause hair to grow back slower
    c. Cause hair to grow back curlier
    d. None of the above

16. What are the three parts of hair?
    a. Cuticle, corium, and papilla
    b. Villa, erector, and lunago
    c. Shaft, body, and cuticle
    d. Follicle, root, and shaft

17. Why is vitamin D a necessity for healthy bones and teeth?
    a. It is needed for the differentiation of osteoclasts to osteoblasts
    b. It is needed for calcium absorption in the intestine
    c. It is needed for fighting gingivitis and calcium buildup
    d. It is not a necessity

18. What degree is a sunburn?
    a. First
    b. Second
    c. Third
    d. Fourth

19. Which of the following layers of skin is the deepest?
    a. Hypodermis
    b. Dermis
    c. Corium
    d. Epidermis

20. Which of the following cells pull the edges of a wound together?
    a. Red blood cells
    b. Melanocytes
    c. Fibroblasts
    d. Osteocytes

21. What role do white blood cells have in wound healing?
    a. Clotting and secreting meshlike barrier
    b. Dissolving debris by chemically breaking bond and mechanically pushing debris to the surface
    c. Fighting infection
    d. Blood thinning

22. Which of the following statements is true about melanin, melanocytes, and skin color?
    a. Adult humans, despite race or gender, have the same amount of melanocytes per skin square inch; skin color difference is due to the amount of melanin secreted from the standard number of melanocytes
    b. Adult humans are beautifully diverse; different skin colors and tones are due to different amounts and arrangements of melanocytes
    c. The more melanin produced, the lighter the skin
    d. Melanocyte absolute numbers are inversely proportional to the concentration of melanin in the skin; in other words, the more melanocytes, the less pigment can be secreted and can ultimately survive in the skin

23. A clinician can estimate the extent of the area covered by a burn using what strategy?
    a. Rule of size
    b. Rule of thumb
    c. Rule of nines
    d. Color rule

24. In a condition called cirrhosis, a liver dysfunction, fair skin appears yellow, but in dark skin the yellow may not be evident. Where can the yellow color be seen?
    a. Eyes
    b. Palms
    c. Teeth
    d. Soles

25. Which of the following sweat glands secrete at the hair follicle of sebaceous glands?
    a. Sebaceous
    b. Apocrine
    c. Eccrine
    d. Creatine

MATCHING EXERCISES

Set 1

_____ 1. Bilirubin   a. Yellow jaundice

_____ 2. Keratin   b. Cools the body

_____ 3. Fibroblasts   c. Sexual attractant

_____ 4. Lipocytes   d. Fat

_____ 5. Sebum   e. Oil

_____ 6. Carotene   f. True skin

_____ 7. Melanin   g. Found in hair and nails

_____ 8. Corium   h. Skin healing

_____ 9. Apocrine   i. Darkening of the skin

_____ 10. Eccrine   j. Natural yellow hue to the skin

Set 2

_____ 1. Cuticle
_____ 2. Dermis
_____ 3. Sebaceous
_____ 4. Lunula
_____ 5. Sudoriferous
_____ 6. Stratum basale
_____ 7. Subcutaneous
_____ 8. Epidermis
_____ 9. Hair follicle
_____ 10. Arrector pili

a. Hypodermis
b. Encloses hair root
c. Upper skin layer of growth
d. Lubricates and moisturizes hair and skin
e. Normally seen layer of skin
f. Contractile tissue associated with hair follicle
g. Covers nail root
h. Contains glands, vessels, collagen, and elastin fibers
i. Excrete water and nitrogenous wastes
j. Proximal, whitish, half-moon part of nail

Set 3

_____ 1. Freckles
_____ 2. Acne
_____ 3. Urticaria
_____ 4. Psoriasis
_____ 5. Fever blister
_____ 6. Shingles
_____ 7. Decubitis ulcer
_____ 8. Abrasion
_____ 9. Ulcer
_____ 10. Malignant melanoma

a. Herpes zoster
b. Patches of excessive melanin production
c. Herpes simplex
d. Cancer
e. Hives
f. Open necrotic sore
g. Itching, scaling, redness, circular borders
h. Bed sores
i. Rubbing off or scratching off of the skin
j. Infection of the sebaceous gland

FILL IN THE BLANK

1. Located in the secondmost deep layer of the skin, _____ fibers help the skin flex with the movement of the body.

2. The most dangerous and life threatening of the skin cancers is _____.

3. Shingles, caused by the _____ virus, are found mainly on the torso or trunk of the body.

4. The skin muscles that contract, indirectly forming what is commonly known as goose flesh, are clinically called _____.

5. The _____ layer of the epidermis is constantly shedding as a part of the skin replacement process.

6. The clinical term for pimple is _____.

7. A human adult, having thousands of sweat glands per square inch, has the potential of excreting up to _____ liters of sweat in 24 hours.

8. Normally it takes _____ seconds to re-perfuse the nail bed when assessing perfusion of the extremity by squeezing the nail.

9. When a person suffers an injury that does not break the skin yet damages the underlying small blood vessels, this person has suffered a _____.

10. "Dry skin" refers to the lack of _____.

11. The most severe of the burns, _____ degree burn, is marked by tissue damage from the skin's surface to the bone.

12. The patient has suffered _____ percent body-surface-area damage when both right upper and lower limbs, the neck, and the head are burned.

13. Nails grow from the nail _____.

14. The substance or pigment responsible for the darkening of the skin is _____.

15. In hepatitis, a liver disease, _____ builds up in the blood, giving the skin an unhealthy yellowish color.

SHORT ANSWER

1. How does "goose flesh" assist in warming the body?

   _____

   _____

   _____

   _____

2. Contrast the three types of skin cancers in terms of severity and depth.

   _____

   _____

   _____

   _____

3. How do bed sores develop?

   _____

   _____

   _____

   _____

4. Besides vitamin D production, what are three functions of skin?

_____

_____

_____

_____

5. What kind of substances can be detected by forensic analysis of the hair?

_____

_____

_____

_____

LABELING ACTIVITY

Label and color code the various structures of the skin using Figure 7–1 on page 151 of your textbook as a guide.

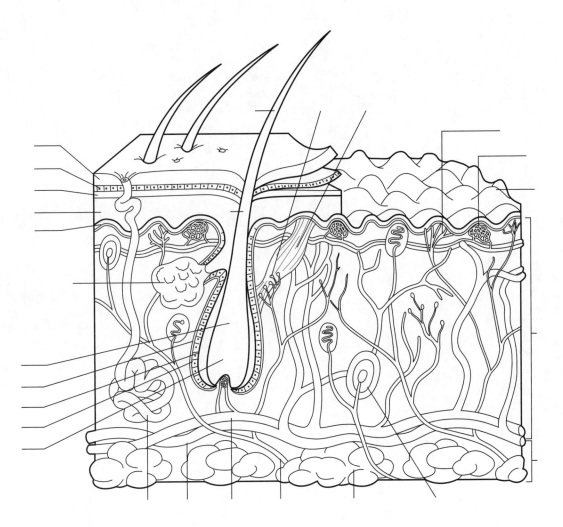

THE NERVOUS SYSTEM: THE BODY'S CONTROL CENTER, PART ONE

Chapter 8

MULTIPLE CHOICE

1. The function of the lateral horn:
   a. Fusing the spinal nerves
   b. Autonomic nervous system
   c. Communication between multipolar motor neurons and bipolar motor neurons
   d. Superhighway for myelinated neurons up and down the spinal cord

2. What are lumbar, sacral, and coccygeal spinal nerves that look like a horse's tail and extend laterally away from a very small area, then route their fibers downward?
   a. Equinal ropa
   b. Cauda equina
   c. Equine threades
   d. Linea alba

3. What two structures make up the entire central nervous system?
   a. Spinal cord and spinal nerve
   b. Gray and white matter
   c. Brain and spinal cord
   d. Brachial and lumbar plexi

4. Both sets of spinal roots fuse to form:
   a. Spinal cord
   b. Spinal nerve
   c. Ganglion
   d. Conus medullaris

5. The terminal vesicle chemicals that inhibit the release of pain neurotransmitter:
   a. Calcium
   b. Serotonin
   c. Sarin
   d. Endorphin

6. Where does the spinal cord end?
   a. Lumbar 2
   b. Coccygeal 3
   c. Plexus 5
   d. Medulla

7. The dorsal horn of the spinal cord is involved with:
   a. Production of cerebral spinal fluid
   b. Motor function
   c. Sensory function
   d. Coordination

8. Choose the correct order of the CNS's protective membrane from inner-most to outermost layer.
   a. Pia mater, dura mater, arachnoid
   b. Arachnoid, dura mater, pia mater
   c. Pia mater, arachnoid, dura mater
   d. Dura mater, arachnoid, pia mater

9. Severe damage to the spinal cord at the lumbar level may result in:
   a. Quadriplegia
   b. Blindness
   c. Bipedalism
   d. Paraplegia

10. How many nerves enter and exit at the cervical region?
    a. 31
    b. 6
    c. 24
    d. 8

11. In the CNS, the glial cells that cover and line cavities:
    a. Ependymal
    b. Oligodendrocytes
    c. Schwann
    d. Astrocytes

12. How many pairs of spinal nerves does the average child have between 13 and 18 years of age?
    a. 31
    b. 29
    c. 17
    d. 24

13. The combination of axon terminal and receiving muscle cell is called:
    a. Nodes of Ranvier
    b. Dendrite
    c. Neuromuscular synapse
    d. Cordae tendinae

14. Which of the following is the part of the neuron that functions in cell metabolism?
    a. Axon terminal
    b. Cell body
    c. Vesicle
    d. Sympathetic

15. The nervous system has an output side called:
    a. Motor
    b. Sensory

c. Parasympathetic

d. Neuroglia

16. Besides the size of the axon, what other characteristic is a determinant in impulse speed at the axon site?

    a. The concentration of the neurotransmitter

    b. Dendritic branches

    c. Myelination

    d. Lack of dendritic branches

17. For repolorization to occur, which of the following is true about movement of ions?

    a. Potassium moves out of cells

    b. Calcium moves into cell

    c. Sodium moves into cell

    d. Chlorine moves out of cell

18. Which of the following vesicle chemicals can be found in the CNS, PNS, and mainly at skeletal neuromuscular synapses?

    a. Norepinephrine

    b. Acetylcholine

    c. Epinephrine

    d. Serotonin

19. Between each Schwann cell, for example, are bare spots where channels must open in order for action potential to flow down the axon with haste. What are they called?

    a. Nodes of Ranvier

    b. Conus medullaris

    c. Myelin

    d. Spudus impulsasis

20. Which of the following axon characteristics will constitute the slowest ionic flow?

    a. wide, myelinated

    b. narrow, unmyelinated

    c. wide, unmyelinated

    d. narrow, myelinated

21. Which of the following systems controls smooth muscle, cardiac muscle, and glands?

    a. Somatic nervous system

    b. Sensory system

    c. Autonomic nervous system

    d. All of the above

22. Which of the following branches in the body's alert system is commonly known as "fight-or-flight"?

    a. Sympathetic

    b. Parasympathetic

    c. Central nervous system

    d. a and b

23. The part of the neuron that functions to receive information from other cells or the environment:
    a. Axon
    b. Vesicle
    c. Dendrite
    d. Schwann

24. Multipolar neurons:
    a. Many cell bodies; single dendrite, single axon
    b. Unlimited ionic transferability
    c. Many dendrites, single axon
    d. One dendrite, multiple axons

25. With a neuron at rest, which of the following is true about the charges inside and outside the cell?
    a. Inside the cell has a positive charge, while outside has a negative charge
    b. Both inside and outside the cell have positive charges
    c. Inside the cell has a negative charge, while outside the cell has a positive charge
    d. Both inside and outside the cell have negative charges

MATCHING EXERCISES

Set 1

_____ 1. Meningitis

_____ 2. Polarized

_____ 3. Botulism

_____ 4. Guillain-Barré syndrome

_____ 5. Paralyzed diaphragm

_____ 6. Multiple sclerosis

_____ 7. Diabetes and alcoholism

_____ 8. Myasthenia gravis

_____ 9. Polio and shingles

_____ 10. Carpal tunnel syndrome

a. Paralysis of four chambers of the heart

b. Systemic, may cause peripheral neuropathy

c. Inflammation of the peripheral nerves leading to rapid onset of paralysis (no known cause)

d. Caused by ingested bacteria, resulting in paralysis

e. Autoimmune disorder in which acetylcholine receptors are reduced

f. Leads to respiratory arrest

g. Flexor tendon sheath becomes inflamed, compressing a wrist nerve

h. Infections that may cause peripheral neuropathy

i. Viral or bacterial infection of the lining of the brain and spinal cord

j. Not stimulated; not excited

k. Damage to the myelin sheath, leading to poor impulse conductivity

Set 2

_____ 1. Neuron
_____ 2. Astrocytes
_____ 3. Satellite cells
_____ 4. Dura mater
_____ 5. Microglia
_____ 6. Arachnoid mater
_____ 7. Schwann
_____ 8. Oligodendrocyte
_____ 9. Pia mater
_____ 10. Ependymal

a. Precursor of the neuroglial cells
b. Metabolic and structural support cells of CNS
c. Support cells of PNS
d. Nerve cells for functional control of the nervous system
e. Covers and lines cavities of the CNS
f. Innermost meningeal layer
g. Outermost meningeal layer
h. Middle meningeal layer
i. Cells that remove debris from the CNS
j. Makes myelin for the CNS
k. Makes myelin for the PNS

Set 3

_____ 1. Endorphin
_____ 2. Acetylcholine
_____ 3. Serotonin
_____ 4. Norepinephrine
_____ 5. Tetrodotoxin
_____ 6. Calcium
_____ 7. Potassium
_____ 8. Sarin
_____ 9. Epidural
_____ 10. Sodium

a. Inhibits acetylcholinesterase; used by terrorist on Tokyo's subways
b. Between dura mater and the vertebral column
c. Triggers the release of neurotransmitters from the vesicles
d. Inhibits the release of pain neurotransmitters
e. Skeletal neuromuscular functional neurotransmitter
f. Poison in fugu
g. Regulate temperature, mood, and onset of sleep
h. Cardiac neuromuscular junctional neurotransmitters
i. Rushes out of cells for repolorization to occur
j. Rushes into the cell for depolorization

FILL IN THE BLANK

1. The parasympathetic division of the nervous system is often called the _____ system.

2. The combination of axon terminal and receiving neural dendrite is called _____.

3. The vesicles at the axon terminal are filled with chemicals called _____.

4. The three horns of the spinal cord are the _____, the _____, and the _____ horns.

5. During labor, a woman may ask for an injection of local anesthesia called a(n) _____, which is administered between the vertebrae and the _____.

6. The spinal cord is divided in half by a(n) _____ and a(n) _____.

7. A pointed structure called the _____ marks the end of the spinal cord.

8. The _____ root is sensory, where the _____ root is motor nerve.

9. The simplest form of motor output that protects us from harm is our _____.

10. In carpal tunnel syndrome, the _____ nerve is affected due to swelling at the wrist.

11. The _____ reflex causes us to respond to loud sound, the _____ reflex involves reaction to sudden intense pain, and the _____ reflex keeps us vertical.

12. The three-layered protective membrane of both the spinal cord and brain is called the _____.

13. A nerve cell is said to be _____ when it is stimulated.

14. When a nerve cell is stimulated, _____ ions rush into the cell.

15. A disorder called _____ is marked by myelin destruction in various areas of the body.

SHORT ANSWER

1. What and where is the cauda equina?

_____

_____

_____

_____

2. What is the stimulation-and-response mechanism of the knee-jerk response?

_____

_____

_____

_____

3. What is the stimulation/depolarization principle of local potential?

_____

_____

_____

_____

4. What area and structures constitute the peripheral nervous system?

_____

_____

_____

_____

5. What is the primary difference between action potential and local potential?

_____

_____

_____

_____

LABELING ACTIVITY

Label the magnified parts of the nervous system using Figure 4–10 on page 83 of your textbook as a guide.

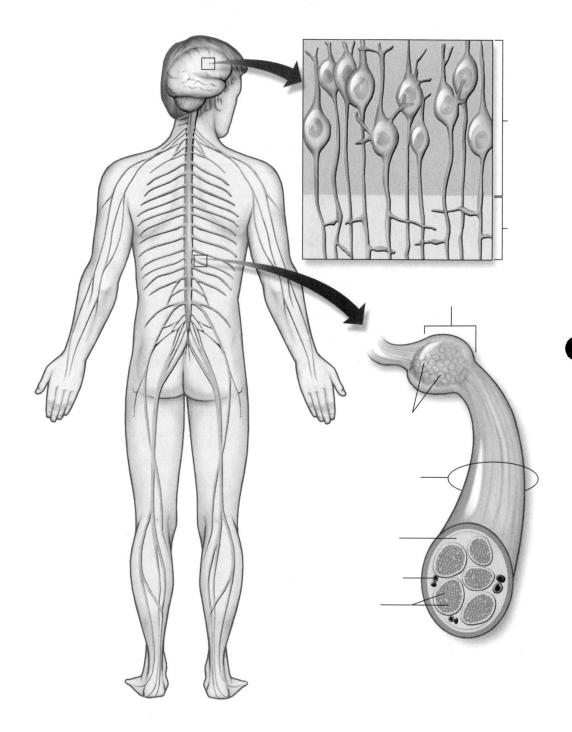

THE NERVOUS SYSTEM: THE BODY'S CONTROL CENTER, PART TWO

Chapter 9

MULTIPLE CHOICE

1. The area of the cerebral cortex that allows understanding and interpretation of somatic sensory information:
   a. Somatic sensory association area
   b. Precentral gyrus
   c. Diencephalon
   d. Limbic reticular formation

2. The map size in the motor cortex is proportional to:
   a. The amount of movement control
   b. The size of the structure
   c. The blood supply
   d. The insula

3. The limbic system is located:
   a. Along craniosacral divisions of the spinal cord
   b. In the cerebellum
   c. In the cerebrum
   d. In the medulla

4. If you violently stub your toe (pain), which of the following pathways carries the information to the brain?
   a. Dorsal column tract
   b. Spinothalamic tract
   c. Spinocerebellar
   d. Spinobulbar

5. Which of the following cranial nerves innervate the skeletal muscles that move the eyeballs?
   a. Trochlear
   b. Abducens
   c. Optic
   d. a and b

6. Where is the arbor vitae located?
   a. The pons
   b. The cerebrum
   c. The midbrain
   d. The cerebellum

7. How many pairs of cranial nerves do we have?
   a. 5
   b. 7
   c. 12
   d. 31

8. The diencephalon is made up of which of the following structures?
   a. Pineal, hypothalamus, pituitary gland, and thalamus
   b. Midbrain, cerebellum, pituitary, and corpus callosum
   c. Midbrain, thalamus, hypothalamus, and cerebellum
   d. Pineal, pituitary, adrenal gland, and midbrain

9. What do the parasympathetic postganglionic neurons and the sympathetic preganglionic neurons secrete?
   a. Norepinephrine / epinephrine
   b. Acetylcholine / acetylcholine
   c. Epinephrine/ acetylcholine
   d. Acetylcholine/ norepinephrine

10. The parietal lobes are mainly responsible for:
    a. Motor activities
    b. Sense perception
    c. Vision
    d. Integration of emotions

11. How many frontal lobes do humans have?
    a. 1
    b. 2
    c. 2 pairs
    d. 4 pairs

12. Where is cerebral spinal fluid made?
    a. In the arachnoid and subdural and central canals by the pituitary glands
    b. In the fourth ventricle by the cerebral aqueduct
    c. In the lateral ventricle(s) by the choroid plexus
    d. In the hypothalamus by the thalamal peptides

13. What separates the frontal lobe from the rest of the brain?
    a. The insula
    b. Central sulcus
    c. Lateral fissure
    d. Latitudinal fissure

14. What separates the parietal lobe(s) from the occipital lobe(s)?
    a. Posterior fissure
    b. Latitudinal fissure
    c. Insula
    d. No obvious dividing line

15. The function of the cerebellum is:
    a. Reflex center for cough and sneeze
    b. Motor coordination and balance
    c. Coordinates heart rate with breathing rate
    d. Interpretation of crude touch and temperature

16. Where is the cerebellum?
    a. Inferior to the medulla
    b. Posterior to the brain stem
    c. Between the thalamus and hypothalamus
    d. Superior to the midbrain

17. The function of the midbrain is:
    a. Coordination
    b. Two-way conduction system pathway to relay visual and auditory impulses
    c. Wisdom, moderation of impulse, and conscience
    d. Production of cerebral spinal fluid

18. Where is the pineal body/gland located?
    a. Posterior to the thalamus between the corpus callosum and cerebellum
    b. Inferior to the cerebellum between the medulla and the pons
    c. Between the cerebrum and the corpus callosum
    d. Anterior and inferior to the hypothalamus

19. Ventricles of the brain are:
    a. Networks of associative neurons that link all four named lobes to each other
    b. Hollows or spaces in the brain for sound resonance and to make the brain lighter
    c. Ridges and crevices on the surface of the brain
    d. Fluid-filled cavities

20. Where is the third ventricle?
    a. Between the cerebrum and the brain stem
    b. In the cerebrum between the frontal and parietal lobes
    c. In the cerebrum spanning the temporal, frontal and parietal lobes
    d. Between the cerebellum and the medulla

21. What may cause CSF to accumulate in the brain?
    a. Blockage of passages between the cavities in the brain
    b. Tumors
    c. Decreased reabsorption
    d. All of the above

22. What effect does acetylcholine have on visceral muscles?
    a. No effect
    b. Inhibits
    c. Excites
    d. Harms

23. The smell of citrus causes Mary to feel anxious. When Mary was a child, her grandmother, who was verbally abusive, served fresh orange juice in the morning before her predictable morning tantrum. What system of the brain coordinates emotion and sense of smell as well as retrieves memories?
    a. Limbic
    b. Sympathetic
    c. Parasympathetic
    d. Somatic sensory

24. Where are the parasympathetic ganglia located?
    a. In the thoracic and lumbar segments of the spinal cord
    b. In the cranial and sacral segments of the spinal cord
    c. Close to the visceral or glandular organs they affect
    d. Running parallel to the vertebral column/spinal cord

25. Where are the sympathetic preganglionic neurons located?
    a. In the thoracic and lumbar segments of the spinal cord
    b. In the cranial and sacral segments of the spinal cord
    c. Close to the visceral or glandular organs they affect
    d. Running parallel to the vertebral column/spinal cord

MATCHING EXERCISES

Set 1

_____ 1. Persistent vegetative state (PVS)

_____ 2. Parasympathetic

_____ 3. Meningitis

_____ 4. Hydrocephalus

_____ 5. Cerebral vascular accident (CVA)

_____ 6. Sympathetic

_____ 7. Flaccid paralysis

_____ 8. Huntington disease

_____ 9. Cerebral palsy

_____ 10. Spastic paralysis

a. Thoracolumbar

b. Hypertonia

c. Nonprogressive childhood disease marked by motor deficits

d. Hypotonia

e. Severe brain injury with an intact brain stem

f. Dysfunction in which nonsterile water seeps into the brain

g. Blood accumulation superficial to the arachnoid

h. Inflammation of the brain and spinal cord covering

i. Hereditary disorder marked by loss of cognitive function

j. Stroke

k. Craniosacral

l. Increased accumulation of CSF in the ventricles

Set 2

_____ 1. Medulla	a. Secretes epinephrine
_____ 2. Parietal lobes	b. Connect left and right hemispheres
_____ 3. Hypothalamus	c. Primary area for hearing function
_____ 4. Pineal gland	d. Primary area for motor function
_____ 5. Frontal lobe	e. Divides the brain into hemispheres
_____ 6. Cerebellum	f. Primary area for vision functions
_____ 7. Corpus callosum	g. Coordination
_____ 8. Temporal lobe	h. Relays sensory and motor information
_____ 9. Pons	i. Regulates heart rate, blood pressure, vomiting
_____ 10. Occipital lobes	j. Regulate body temperature, fear, and pleasure
	k. Secretes melatonin
	l. Primary area for sensory functions

Set 3

_____ 1. Facial nerve	a. Vision
_____ 2. Oculomotor nerve	b. Movement of the eye, C. N. IV
_____ 3. Glossopharyngeal nerve	c. Sensation of the face and muscles for chewing
_____ 4. Accessory nerve	d. Muscles of expression like squinting and smiling
_____ 5. Olfactory nerve	e. Smell
_____ 6. Trochlear nerve	f. Swallowing and taste, C. N. IX
_____ 7. Optic nerve	g. Movement of the tongue
_____ 8. Hypoglossal nerve	h. Movement of the shoulder's trapezius muscles
_____ 9. Trigeminal nerve	i. Movement of the eye, C. N. III
_____ 10. Vagus nerve	j. Sensation of the stomach (bellyache)
	k. Hearing and balance

FILL IN THE BLANK

1. From the outside, you can see that the brain consists of three parts; the
_____, _____, and
_____.

2. The right and left hemispheres of the brain are divided by the
_____ fissure.

3. The surface of the cerebrum has broken ridges called

   _____.

4. The two cranial nerves involved in taste are the _____ and the _____ nerves.

5. The occipital lobes are responsible for _____.

6. The dividing line called the _____ separates the temporal lobe from the rest of the brain.

7. The three sections of the brain stem are the _____, the _____, and the _____.

8. The layer of gray matter surrounding the white matter of the brain is called _____.

9. The insula is located deep within the _____ of the brain.

10. The ventricles of the brain contain _____.

11. Position and postural sensory information is carried in the _____ pathway of the somatic sensory system.

12. The sympathetic division of the autonomic nervous system stimulates the _____ gland to secrete epinephrine.

13. A remarkable woman named Harriet Tubman was born into slavery but had the courage to free herself, hundreds of kidnapped Africans, and their descendants. Ironically, considering that she was constantly and dangerously on the run, she suffered from narcolepsy, which means she would fall asleep uncontrollably. As a child, due to a violent blow by the plantation overseer, Harriet Tubman's _____ of the brain was damaged. This part of the brain is vital in the maintenance of conscious awareness.

14. Of the two divisions of the autonomic nervous system, the _____ controls the fight-or-flight response.

15. The corticospinal and corticobulbar tracts carry _____ signals to synaptic junctions in the ventral horn of the spinal cord.

SHORT ANSWER

1. What is meant by *contralateral* information entering and leaving the brain?

   _____

   _____

   _____

   _____

2. Why is the epidural space absent in the brain?

   _____

   _____

   _____

   _____

3. What is the purpose of brain convolutions?

   _____

   _____

   _____

   _____

4. Besides location, what are two differences between the spinal nerves and the cranial nerves?

   _____

   _____

   _____

   _____

5. What effects do both the sympathetic and parasympathetic nervous systems have on skeletal muscle, cardiac muscle, and the muscle surrounding the digestive tract?

   _____

   _____

   _____

   _____

LABELING ACTIVITY

Identify the following structures. Then color code the following brain regions: cerebral cortex, interior cerebrum, diencephalon, midbrain, pons, medulla oblongata using Figure 9–3 on page 202 of your textbook as a guide.

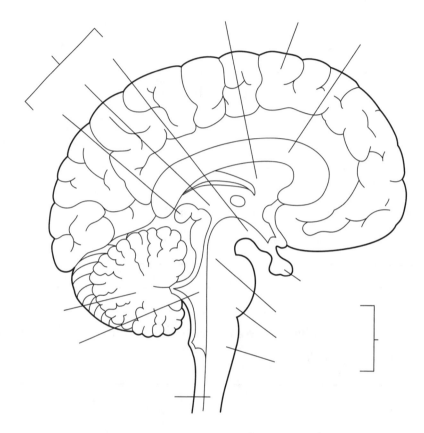

THE ENDOCRINE SYSTEM: THE BODY'S OTHER CONTROL CENTER

Chapter 10

MULTIPLE CHOICE

1. What is the target organ(s) for glucagon?
   a. Pancreas
   b. Kidneys
   c. Adrenals
   d. Liver

2. How do hormones and neurotransmitters (NT) differ?
   a. Hormones are secreted by exocrine glands, and NTs are secreted from endocrine glands
   b. Hormones are fast to take action, and NTs are slow to take effect
   c. Hormones are secreted by endocrine glands, and NTs are secreted from axon terminals
   d. b and c

3. Where are the adrenal glands located?
   a. Above the kidneys
   b. In the brain stem
   c. In the chest
   d. In the neck

4. Which feedback mechanism does insulin operate on?
   a. Positive
   b. Negative
   c. Neutral
   d. Neural

5. Which hormone needs iodine for production?
   a. Insulin
   b. Thymosin
   c. Iodomelanoin
   d. Thyroxine

6. Which gland or organ secretes releasing and inhibitory hormones controlling the master gland?
   a. Pituitary
   b. Adrenal
   c. Pancreas
   d. Hypothalamus

7. Where is the pancreas located?
   a. In the abdomen
   b. In the brain
   c. In the neck
   d. In the pelvis

8. What directly influences the production of testosterone?
   a. Gonadotropin-releasing hormone
   b. Corticotropic hormone
   c. Luteinizing hormone
   d. ACTH

9. What gland is at its greatest size and efficiency in childhood fighting infection and helps in the maturation of white blood cells?
   a. Thyroid
   b. Thymus
   c. Testis
   d. Adrenals

10. Which of the following is a function of one of the hormones secreted by the adrenal cortex?
    a. Fright and flight
    b. Salt and fluid balance
    c. Skin pigmentation
    d. Iodine production

11. What is the target organ for ACTH?
    a. Adrenals
    b. Adenoids
    c. Anterior pituitary
    d. Arterial walls

12. What is true about hormones?
    a. Focuses on targets very close
    b. Affect a single cell
    c. Effects wear off quickly
    d. Effects are long lasting

13. Why are steroid hormones so powerful?
    a. Steroid hormones pass easily through the target cell membrane and interact with the cell's DNA
    b. They are always secreted in great amounts
    c. They interact with the neuronal cell bodies as well as the neural membranes
    d. All of the above

14. What is the target organ for ADH?
    a. Adenoids
    b. Kidneys
    c. Adrenals
    d. Pancreas

15. Which hormone antagonizes glucagon?
    a. Insulin
    b. Glycogen
    c. Thymosin
    d. Calcitonin

16. Where is the pineal gland located?
    a. In the chest
    b. In the pelvis
    c. In the neck
    d. In the brain

17. What may occur if calcitonin is hypersecreted?
    a. Low blood calcium
    b. High blood cholesterol
    c. Low blood sugar
    d. High blood viscosity

18. Where is melanocyte-stimulating hormone produced?
    a. Posterior pituitary
    b. Thyroid
    c. Parathyroid
    d. Anterior pituitary

19. Which gland is located in the chest?
    a. Thyroid
    b. Thymus
    c. Pineal
    d. Pituitary

20. The diencephalon is home to the:
    a. Hypothalamus
    b. Adrenals
    c. Thymus
    d. Pancreas

21. Which hormone increases the release of LH and FSH from its releasing gland?
    a. Adrenocorticotropic hormone
    b. Estrogen
    c. Adrenocorticosteroids
    d. Gonadotropin-releasing hormone

22. Parathyroid hormone targets:
    a. Bladder
    b. Skin
    c. Bone
    d. Mammary glands (breasts)

23. Polyuria (increased urination) is a symptom of:
    a. Addison disease
    b. Diabetes mellitus
    c. Cushing disease
    d. Hashimoto disease

24. For uterine contraction during childbirth the expectant mother needs to secrete:
    a. Iodine
    b. Estrogen
    c. Oxytocin
    d. Prolactin

25. A tumor of the adrenal gland resulting in excess secretion of epinephrine:
    a. Hashimoto disease
    b. Pheochromocytoma
    c. Addison disease
    d. Diabetes mellitus

MATCHING EXERCISES

Set 1

Match the gland to the hormone it produces

_____ 1. Pineal	a. Antidiuretic hormone
_____ 2. Anterior pituitary	b. Thyroxine
_____ 3. Posterior pituitary	c. Melanocyte-stimulating hormone
_____ 4. Ovaries	d. Progesterone
_____ 5. Pancreas	e. Testosterone
_____ 6. Thymus	f. Melatonin
_____ 7. Testis	g. Insulin
_____ 8. Adrenal medulla	h. Thymosin
_____ 9. Hypothalamus	i. None
_____ 10. Thyroid	j. Epinephrine

Set 2

Match the hormone to its action

_____ 1. Parathyroid hormone	a. Increases blood glucose
_____ 2. Luteinizing hormones	b. Ovulation
_____ 3. Follicle-stimulating hormone	c. Decreases blood calcium
	d. Decreases blood sugar
_____ 4. Triiodothyronine	e. Regulates secondary sexual characteristics
_____ 5. Oxytocin	
_____ 6. Calcitonin	f. Increases blood calcium
_____ 7. Insulin	g. Increases metabolism; secreted by gland located in neck
_____ 8. Norepinephrine	
_____ 9. Melatonin	h. Triggers sleep
_____ 10. Adrenocorticosteroids	i. Milk ejection
	j. Prolongs fight-or-flight response
	k. Regulates sperm and egg production

Set 3

_____ 1. Cushing

_____ 2. Addison

_____ 3. Diabetes mellitus

_____ 4. Dwarfism

_____ 5. Bone deterioration

_____ 6. Testicular shrinkage

_____ 7. Graves' disease

_____ 8. Decreased milk production

_____ 9. Impaired ovulation

_____ 10. Hashimoto disease

a. Steroid abuse

b. Upper body obesity; high blood sugar

c. Decrease in insulin production or recognition

d. Hyposecretion of prolactin

e. Swollen thyroid gland; hypothyroidism

f. Decreased luteinizing hormone

g. Decreased growth hormone during childhood

h. Hypersecretion of parathyroid hormone

i. Weight loss; low BP; insufficient cortisol

j. Hyperthyroidism; bulging eyes

FILL IN THE BLANK

1. In females, _____ stimulates the smooth muscle tissue in the wall of uterus, promoting labor and delivery.

2. Another name for the anterior pituitary glands is _____.

3. The _____ is embedded in the mediastinum, posterior to the sternum.

4. The pancreas secretes _____ and _____.

5. A hyposecretion of cortisol _____.

6. T3 and T4 secretions are controlled by _____ secreted by the anterior pituitary.

7. Milk production is controlled by the hormone _____ and milk ejection is controlled by a hormone _____.

8. The hypothalamus regulates the release of hormones from the _____ gland.

9. MSH from the pituitary gland targets _____.

10. Both alcohol and coffee inhibit the hormone _____.

11. The three ways hormone levels are regulated are _____, _____, and _____.

12. Prednisone mimics the hormones secreted by the _____.

13. The antagonist hormone to calcitonin is secreted by the
    _____ gland.

14. _____ are chemical messengers that are released in
    one tissue and transported by the bloodstream to affect target cells and
    other tissues.

15. The hormone unique to females is _____.

SHORT ANSWER

1. Explain the functional difference between an exocrine gland and an
   endocrine gland.

   _____

   _____

   _____

   _____

2. What are two mutual side effects or risk factors with anabolic steroid
   abuse in both men and women?

   _____

   _____

   _____

   _____

3. Why do alcohol and coffee increase urine output?

   _____

   _____

   _____

   _____

4. What is meant by *humoral* control of hormonal levels?

   _____

   _____

   _____

   _____

5. What sort of interaction do steroid hormones have on target cells so that
   the cells will demonstrate a change in function?

   _____

   _____

   _____

   _____

LABELING ACTIVITY

Name the pictured glands using Figure 4–11 on page 84 of your textbook as a guide.

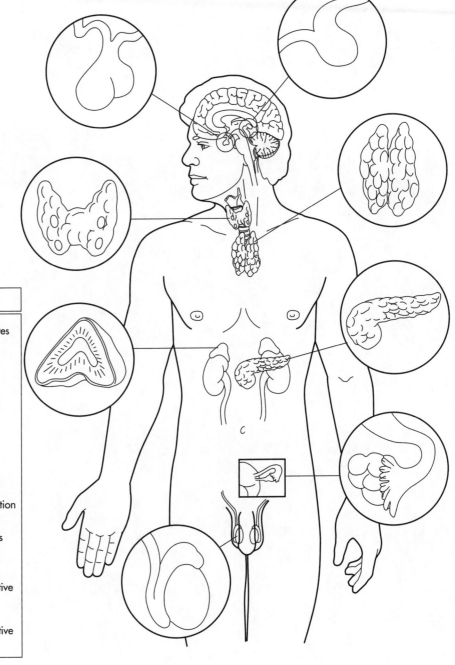

Organ	Primary Functions
Pituitary Gland	Controls other glands, regulates growth and fluid balance
Thyroid Gland	Controls tissue metabolic rate and regulates calcium levels
Parathyroid Gland	Regulates calcium levels (with thyroid)
Thymus	Controls white blood cell maturation
Adrenal Glands	Adjust water balance, tissue metabolism, cardiovascular and respiratory activity
Kidneys	Control red blood cell production and elevate blood pressure
Pancreas	Regulates blood glucose levels
Gonads	
Testes	Support male sexual characteristics and reproductive functions
Ovaries	Support female sexual characteristics and reproductive functions

THE SPECIAL SENSES: THE SIGHTS AND SOUNDS

Chapter 11

MULTIPLE CHOICE

1. Which of the following correctly describes *phantom* pain?
   a. Pain at the location where a vital organ was recently removed
   b. Pain that originates in one part of the body but is felt in another
   c. Pain that is mysteriously felt in the daytime but is elusive at nighttime
   d. Pain felt in a limb that was amputated

2. Umami:
   a. Ringing in the ears
   b. Shadows in the visual spectrum
   c. Sporadic deafness and loss of equilibrium
   d. Taste of glutamates

3. Which of the following is *not* a special sense?
   a. Sight
   b. Sound
   c. Hunger
   d. Smell

4. How does the body rid itself of excess tears that are normally produced?
   a. The eyeball itself has the capacity to reabsorb the tears back into the aqueous humor
   b. With each and every blink, the eyelid collects the tears and directs it to the back of the orbit
   c. The face vasoconstricts its blood vessels, which increases the temperature of the eyeball and surrounding structures, and in turn evaporates the tears
   d. Excess tears drain into the nose via two small holes in the inner corner of the eye

5. Which of the following is true about the rods and cones?
   a. There are far more rods than cones
   b. There are far more cones that rods
   c. There are equal amounts of rods to cones
   d. The number of rods and cones are correctable with prescription eyeglasses

6. What is the primary function of the ossicles?
   a. Amplification of the sound waves that enter the middle ear
   b. Channeling of the sound waves that enter the outer ear
   c. Interpretation of sound waves that enter the inner ear
   d. Vibrates the eardrum

7. Which of the cranial nerves transmit from the cochlea and semicircular canals to the brain?
   a. Cranial nerve VIII
   b. Cranial nerve VI
   c. Abducens
   d. a and c

8. The eyeball sits in a conical cavity called the:
   a. Optic
   b. Orbit
   c. Ocular
   d. Olfactory

9. Which of the following structures function as sensors that activate a shielding effect as foreign objects approach the eyeball?
   a. Pupils
   b. Eyelashes
   c. Lens
   d. Eyebrows

10. Senses such as thirst, nausea, and the need to defecate are what kind of senses?
    a. Special
    b. Cutaneous
    c. Systemic
    d. Visceral

11. Which of the following is not a taste that the tongue's special sense can detect?
    a. Sweet
    b. Spicy
    c. Bitter
    d. Sour

12. Where is the eardrum located?
    a. Between middle and inner ear
    b. Between the middle and outer ear
    c. Between the outer ear and labyrinth
    d. At the outer rim of the external auditory meatus

13. The sense of taste is referred to as:
    a. Olfactory
    b. Gastration
    c. Mechanoreception
    d. Gustatory

14. Arrange the ossicles in the direction that sound waves would travel through them in order to channel and be sent to the brain for interpretation:
    a. Malleus, incus, stapes

b. Hammer, anvil, incus

c. Stirrup, anvil, hammer

d. Incus, malleus, stirrup

15. Which of the three layers of the eyeball is highly vascularized and also contains the iris?

   a. Cornea

   b. Choroid

   c. Retina

   d. Sclera

16. When there is low light, the iris will:

   a. Defer activity to the rods

   b. Tighten

   c. Relax

   d. Rely on the cones

17. The retina continues posteriorly to the back of the eye socket and forms what nerve?

   a. Oculomotor

   b. Optic

   c. Cranial nerve VIII

   d. b and c

18. The function of earwax is to:

   a. Filter sound

   b. Trap foreign particles

   c. Maintain surface tension of the inner ear

   d. Monitor pressure

19. What is the function of the muscles surrounding the lens of the eye?

   a. To alter the shape of the lens, making it either thinner or thicker

   b. To move the eyeball right, left, up, or down depending on the focal point

   c. To decrease or increase the diameter of the iris

   d. To push the lens forward or pull it back depending on the pressure of the fluids of the eye

20. When the iris contracts, what part of the eye changes, and in what way?

   a. Retina becomes wider

   b. Cornea becomes opaque

   c. Pupil becomes larger

   d. Pupil becomes smaller

21. Which one of the following taste receptors is located at the very front or tip of the tongue?

   a. Sour

   b. Bitter

   c. Salty

   d. Sweet

22. Where are the olfactory receptors?

   a. Back of throat

   b. Top of nasal cavity

   c. Sides of tongue

   d. In the organ of Corti

23. When Anne was 9 years old, she started having difficulty seeing the board from the back of the classroom. The teacher did not change the size of her script to warrant this gradual change in visual acuity. It was evident that Anne may be in the early stages of:
    a. Myopia
    b. Glaucoma
    c. Otetis media
    d. Hyperopia

24. Receptors of the skin, which include touch, heat, and pain, are referred to as:
    a. Organ of Corti
    b. Visceral sense
    c. Cutaneous senses
    d. Dermatitis

25. Sound travels best in:
    a. Air at high altitudes
    b. Air at lower altitude
    c. Air at high temperature
    d. Solid or liquid medium

MATCHING EXERCISES

Set 1

_____ 1. Tympanic cavity
_____ 2. Hammer
_____ 3. Stirrup
_____ 4. Pinna
_____ 5. Anvil
_____ 6. Cochlea
_____ 7. Semicircular
_____ 8. Endolymph
_____ 9. Auditory
_____ 10. Acoustic

a. Canal or tube leading from the middle ear to the throat

b. Middle ossicle between the malleus and the stapes

c. Nerve also known as vestibulocochlear

d. Auricle

e. Fluid associated with organ of Corti

f. Ossicle directly against the oval window

g. Ossicle directly against the eardrum

h. Cranial nerve VI

i. Bony spiral structure of the inner ear associated with sound

j. Another name for the middle ear

k. Three canal loops of the inner ear associated more with equilibrium than actual sound

Set 2

_____ 1. Myopia
_____ 2. Labyrinthitis
_____ 3. Tinnitus
_____ 4. Conjunctivitis
_____ 5. Otitis media
_____ 6. Amblyopia
_____ 7. Presbyopia
_____ 8. Cataracts
_____ 9. Glaucoma
_____ 10. Hyperopia

a. Lazy eye
b. Inflammation of the lining of the eye
c. A ringing sound in the ears
d. Inflammation of the inner ear
e. Nearsightedness
f. Loss of taste
g. Farsightedness
h. Farsightedness brought about by age
i. Infection of the middle ear
j. Increased pressure in the fluid of the eye
k. Clouded lens of the eye

Set 3

_____ 1. Rods
_____ 2. Cornea
_____ 3. Cones
_____ 4. Sclera
_____ 5. Lens
_____ 6. Pupil
_____ 7. Lacrimal
_____ 8. Vitreous
_____ 9. Iris
_____ 10. Aqueous

a. Gland that secretes tears
b. Humor that bathes the iris, pupil, and lens
c. Bends light; surrounded by involuntary muscles
d. Clinical term for the entire middle layer of the eyeball
e. Sphincter that controls how much light passes into the eye
f. Humor that occupies the posterior cavity of the eyeball
g. Photoreceptor active in dim light
h. Hole or circular opening in the middle of the sphincter muscle of the eyes
i. Whites of the eye
j. Photoreceptor active in bright light
k. Transparent structure allowing outside light rays into the eye

FILL IN THE BLANK

1. As it is associated with sound, the _____ of the inner ear sends sensory impulses to the _____ of the brain.

2. The inner ear is also called the _____.

3. ESP is the abbreviation for _____.

4. The glands that produce tears are the _____ glands.

5. Brown, hazel, blue, and green eyes are actually colors of the _____ of the eyeball.

6. The fluid that fills the posterior cavity of the eye is called

    _____.

7. Earwax is produced by the _____ gland for the main

    purpose of _____.

8. The vestibule chamber of the ear houses the _____.

9. The part of the external ear that collects and directs sound waves into

    the external auditory meatus is the _____.

10. The eardrum is clinically called the _____ membrane.

11. The two fluids of the inner ear are the _____ and the

    _____.

12. The eustachian tube leads from the ear to the _____ of

    the throat.

13. As it is associated with equilibrium, the _____ of the

    inner ear sends sensory signals to the _____ of the

    brain.

14. An extremely contagious form of conjunctivitis is

    _____.

15. Vision, hearing, and smell are known as _____ senses.

SHORT ANSWER

1. What are the functions of the eyelid?

    _____

    _____

    _____

    _____

2. Explain the phenomenon called *adaptation* as it applies to sensation.

    _____

    _____

    _____

    _____

3. Describe the process of *accommodation* as it applies to the lens of the eye.

    _____

    _____

    _____

    _____

4. What are the three layers of the eyeball?

_____

_____

_____

_____

5. Contrast the three types of auditory conduction.

_____

_____

_____

_____

LABELING ACTIVITY

Label and color the parts of the ear using Figure 11–3 on page 254 of your textbook as a guide.

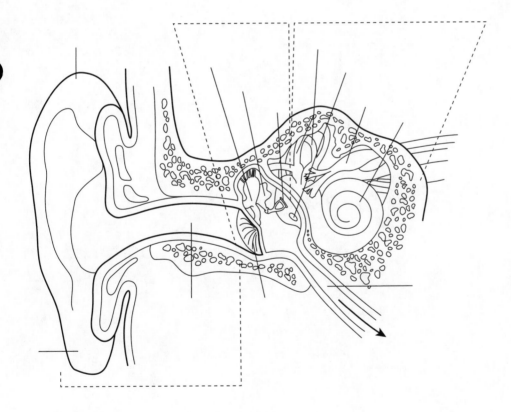

THE CARDIOVASCULAR SYSTEM: TRANSPORT AND SUPPLY

Chapter 12

MULTIPLE CHOICE

1. The white blood cells that produce heparin:
   a. Lymphocytes
   b. Basophils
   c. Eosinophils
   d. Erythrocytes

2. The function of hemoglobin is:
   a. Clotting
   b. Gas transport
   c. Immunity
   d. Production of blood cells

3. Which of the blood types is considered the *universal recipient?*
   a. A
   b. O
   c. B
   d. AB

4. Where in the chest is the heart located?
   a. Directly in the middle of the chest, with apex above the base
   b. Slightly right of center with the base resting on the diaphragm
   c. Half to the right and half to the left of chest midline, with the base directly resting on the diaphragm
   d. Slightly left of center with the base above the apex

5. Which of the following is true about a type B positive person?
   a. It is safe to give blood to a type B positive and O negative
   b. It is safe to give blood to a type B positive and AB positive
   c. It is safe to give blood to a type B positive and O positive
   d. It is safe to receive blood from a type B positive and type AB positive

6. The right side of the heart is responsible for:
   a. Collecting from and distributing both oxygenated and deoxygenated blood to just the right side of the body
   b. Collecting deoxygenated blood from all over the body and sending it just to the lungs
   c. Sending oxygenated blood to the upper body and collecting deoxygenated blood from the lower body
   d. Sending deoxygenated blood to and collecting oxygenated blood from the lungs

7. What type of self-antigens do people with blood type O have?
   a. A antigens
   b. A and B antigens
   c. None
   d. O antigens

8. The left side of the heart is responsible for:
   a. collecting from and distributing deoxygenated blood to just the left side of the body
   b. sending oxygenated blood to the lower body and collecting deoxygenated blood from the upper body
   c. collecting oxygenated blood from the lungs and sending it to the entire body
   d. sending deoxygenated blood to the lungs and collecting similar blood from the head

9. What does serotonin do?
   a. Vasoconstricts
   b. Clots blood
   c. Unclots blood
   d. Increases temperature of the plasma

10. What types of plasma antibodies do people with blood type A have?
    a. A antibodies
    b. B antibodies
    c. O antibodies
    d. A and B antibodies

11. Which of the blood types is considered a *universal donor?*
    a. A
    b. B
    c. O
    d. AB

12. What prevents blood from shooting into the left atrium upon ventricular contraction?
    a. The third chamber, called the atrioventricular chamber
    b. A valve called the tricuspid
    c. A valve called the mitral
    d. Decompression of the diaphragm

13. Which of the following is true in regard to the Rh factor?
    a. If an Rh-positive father and an Rh-negative mother have a child that inherits the father's blood type, it will be healthy, but the second child of the same couple will have complications if he or she is also Rh-positive
    b. If an Rh-negative father and an Rh-positive mother have a child that inherited the father's blood type, then there will be complications with the growth and development of this child
    c. If an Rh-positive father and an Rh-negative mother have a child that inherits the mother's blood type, it will be healthy, but their second child, if Rh-positive, will have complications
    d. If an Rh-positive father and an Rh-positive mother have an obvious Rh-positive child, it will be healthy, but their second child, if Rh-negative, will have complications

14. How does chewing an aspirin tablet help in a heart attack?
    a. It conducts electrical current that gives the heart muscles an instant jolt
    b. It has the ability to vasoconstrict, temporarily raising blood pressure
    c. It has anticoagulating ability to help blood flow easier
    d. It increases RBCs, allowing more oxygen to the heart muscle

15. In measuring blood pressure, inflate the cuff to what measure? Then open the valve slightly so the cuff slowly deflates as you listen to what?
    a. 30 mmHg above the point where you lose the pulse sound/brachial artery
    b. 120 mmHg/radial artery
    c. 120 mmHg above the point where lose the pulse sound/carotid artery
    d. The point where you lose the pulse sound/chest

16. Which of the following statements is true?
    a. The right ventricle sends blood to both the right and left lungs to pick up a fresh supply of oxygen
    b. The left ventricle sends blood to both the right and left lungs to pick up a fresh supply of oxygen
    c. The right ventricle sends blood to the right lung, and left ventricle sends blood to the left lung to pick up a fresh supply of oxygen
    d. The right and left atria direct blood to the right and left lung respectively

17. Which of the heart chambers is the thickest?
    a. Atrioventricular
    b. Left ventricle
    c. Right atria
    d. Left atria

18. Which of the following is true about resting heart rate?
    a. On average, males have a faster rate than females
    b. On average, male and female rates are the same provided that they are the same weight
    c. On average, females have a faster rate than males
    d. There is absolutely no viable evidence that relative resting heart rate is gender specific

19. Correctly arrange the electrical wiring of the heart from where the impulse is initially generated to where it is carried to the contractile muscle cells.
    a. Bundle of His, vagus nerve, sinoatrial node, atrioventricular node
    b. Sinoatrial node, vagus nerve, Purkinje cells, atrioventricular node, bundle of His
    c. Sinoatrial node, atrioventricular node, bundle of His, Purkinje fibers
    d. Vagus nerve, sinoatrial node, atrioventricular node Purkinje fibers, bundle of His

20. On the ECG, which of the waves represents the depolarization of the atria?
    a. T
    b. QRS
    c. It is masked by another wave
    d. P

21. On the ECG, which of the waves represents the repolarization of the ventricles?
    a. T
    b. It is masked by another wave
    c. QRS
    d. P

22. Immediately after the depolarization of the ventricles, what happens?
    a. The atria contract
    b. The atria relax
    c. The ventricles contract
    d. The ventricles relax

23. How much blood do humans normally have?
    a. 1 to 3 liters
    b. 4 to 6 liters
    c. 7 to 9 liters
    d. 11 to 13 liters

24. One of the leukocytes secretes heparin. What does heparin do?
    a. Clots blood
    b. Carries oxygen
    c. Threads a biological net
    d. Keeps blood from clotting

25. Which of the formed elements has the capacity to release serotonin?
    a. Platelets
    b. Basophils
    c. Eosinophils
    d. Neutrophils

MATCHING EXERCISES

Set 1

_____ 1. Monocytes
_____ 2. Phagocytosis
_____ 3. Erythrocytes
_____ 4. Basophils
_____ 5. Leukocytes
_____ 6. Lymphocytes
_____ 7. Hemopoiesis
_____ 8. Neutrophils
_____ 9. Thrombocytes
_____ 10. Eosinophils

a. Produce antibodies
b. The process by which RBCs are created
c. A granulocyte that attempts to destroy bacteria by engulfing
d. WBCs involved in allergies and inflammation
e. WBCs functioning to combat parasites and decrease allergies
f. The process by which a cell surrounds and ingests an invader
g. Collective term for white blood cells
h. Collective term for red blood cells
i. Higher than normal amounts in chronic infections
j. Platelets

Set 2

_____ 1. Agglutination
_____ 2. Pallor
_____ 3. Tunic
_____ 4. Embolus
_____ 5. Inotropism
_____ 6. Node
_____ 7. Anastomoses
_____ 8. Vasoconstriction
_____ 9. Vasodilation
_____ 10. Iron

a. Arterial reaction resulting in increased pressure within the vessel
b. Deficiency may lead to anemia
c. Pale skin
d. Self-antigens on RBC cell surface bind to antibodies, clumping
e. Branching of arteries so there is ample blood supply to the entire heart
f. A surface layer of a blood vessel
g. Results in increased blood vessel diameter
h. Pacemaker
i. Traveling clot
j. Means the force of cardiac contractions
k. Mineral produced by the heart

Set 3

_____ 1. Hemophilia
_____ 2. Cerebral vascular accident
_____ 3. Cor pulmonale
_____ 4. Anemia
_____ 5. Aneurysm
_____ 6. Myocardial infarction
_____ 7. Atherosclerosis
_____ 8. Arteriosclerosis
_____ 9. Leukemia
_____ 10. Valvular insufficiency

a. The right ventricle is not pumping blood efficiently
b. Accumulation of plaque in vessels
c. The mitral valve, may be too large
d. High amounts of immature WBCs
e. Hardening of the blood vessels
f. Uncontrollable bleeding
g. Low amount of viable RBCs
h. Weakening of arterial wall
i. Heart attack
j. Stroke

FILL IN THE BLANK

1. Arteries move blood _____ the heart.

2. The wall that separates the two lower chambers of the heart is called the _____.

3. On the ECG, the wave that represents the depolarization of the ventricles is the _____.

4. Blood transports _____, _____, _____, and _____.

5. Upon separation by centrifugation, blood is seen to have two major components, _____ and _____.

6. In the clotting mechanism, prothrombin, produced by the _____, is converted to thrombin with the help of vitamin _____.

7. The wall that separates the two upper chambers of the heart is called the _____.

8. Blood from the right upper chamber drains through the _____ valve to the lower chamber on the same side.

9. When body temperature increases, the response of the cardiac rate and force is to _____.

10. The SA node is located in/on the _____ of the heart.

11. The electrolyte _____, when at high levels, can prolong heart contractions to the point that the heart can actually stop beating.

12. The biological "net" or "gauze" made of _____ is formed by posttrauma attempts to cover the wound and prevent blood cells from escaping.

13. When examining the plaque removed from a blood vessel, you will find the main component of this substance is _____.

14. Two instruments, the _____ and the _____, are used to determine a patient's or client's blood pressure.

15. The two large vessels that empty into the right atrium are the _____ and the _____.

SHORT ANSWER

1. Contrast the terms *agglutination* and *coagulation*.

_____

_____

_____

_____

2. Explain the exception to the rule that arteries carry oxygenated blood and veins carry deoxygenated blood.

_____

_____

_____

3. Besides water, name four substances that are dissolved in plasma.

_____

_____

_____

_____

4. What effects do the sympathetic and the parasympathetic divisions of the nervous system have on the heart, respectively?

_____

_____

_____

_____

_____

5. How do the walls of the heart receive a blood supply in order to stay healthy?

_____

_____

_____

_____

LABELING ACTIVITY

Label the figure and color the blood vessels using red to indicate oxygenated blood, blue to indicate deoxygenated blood and purple to indicate where the oxygen level changes using Figure 12–1 on page 271 of your textbook as a guide.

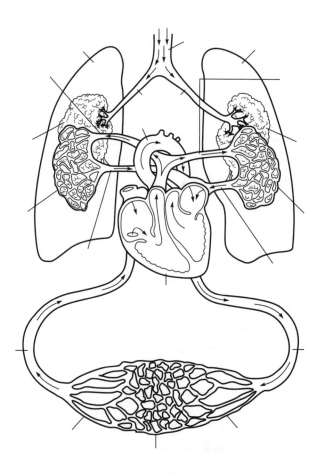

◯ = Blood low in oxygen and high in carbon dioxide (deoxygenated).

◯ = Blood high in oxygen and low in carbon dioxide (oxygenated).

THE RESPIRATORY SYSTEM: IT'S A GAS

Chapter 13

MULTIPLE CHOICE

1. What type of cells make up the membrane that lines the respiratory region of the nose and most of the airway?
   a. Stratified flagellated cuboidal
   b. Simple squamous
   c. Stratified globetulated squamous
   d. Pseudostratified ciliated columnar

2. The region that separates one lung from the other:
   a. Pleura
   b. Mediastinum
   c. Carina
   d. Septum

3. The purpose of pleural fluid is to:
   a. Reduce friction as an individual breathes
   b. Moisten air passage
   c. Filter debris
   d. Reduce surface tension within the bronchioles

4. The main function of surfactant is to:
   a. Nourish the trachea
   b. Reduce friction as a person swallows
   c. Reduce surface tension in the alveoli
   d. Filter gases in the nasal cavity

5. Which of the following statements is/are true about sinuses?
   a. Interconnect with the nasal cavity via small passageways
   b. We are born with three of the four sinuses
   c. The sinuses are filled with air, making the skull heavier and more protective
   d. All of the above

6. Which of the three sections of the pharynx contains the adenoids?
   a. Tracheopharynx
   b. Nasopharynx
   c. Oropharynx
   d. Laryngopharynx

7. Which of the following statements is true about inspiration?
   a. For inspiration to take place, pressure in the thoracic cavity needs to decrease
   b. For inspiration to take place, atmospheric pressure needs to be lower than thoracic pressure
   c. For inspiration to take place, pressure in the thoracic cavity needs to increase
   d. For inspiration to take place, atmospheric pressure and thoracic pressure need to be equal

8. What is the purpose of cilia in the airways?
   a. To propel air into the lungs
   b. To propel trapped debris upward to be expelled from the body
   c. To trap food and prevent entry into the windpipe
   d. For olfaction

9. Which of the three sections of the pharynx conducts air, food, and liquid?
   a. Oropharynx
   b. Nasopharynx
   c. Tracheopharynx
   d. All of the above

10. Which of the three parts of the sternum is fragile and needs to be avoided if performing CPR on a victim?
    a. Manubrium
    b. Body
    c. Hilus
    d. Xiphoid

11. Which of the paired tonsils is located in the middle pharyngeal section?
    a. Adenoid
    b. Palatine
    c. Lingual
    d. Submandibular

12. Directly below the Adam's apple is a large cartilage called the:
    a. carina
    b. alveolus
    c. philus
    d. cricoid

13. How does the epiglottis function in terms of us swallowing and breathing?
    a. As we breathe in, the epiglottis moves from its natural closed position to an open position so air can enter the larynx and trachea
    b. As we swallow, the epiglottis flaps down to close off the larynx so food does not slip into that area
    c. As we breathe in, the epiglottis closes off our esophagus so air does not enter into that area
    d. It acts as a "guard gate," closing off the eustachian tubes so air and food cannot enter and cause problems

14. The name of the membrane that covers or wraps each lung:
    a. Pulmonary sheath
    b. Synovial membrane
    c. Visceral pleura
    d. Parietal aponeurosis

15. The function of the conchae is to:
    a. Warm and moisten air
    b. Filter large particles
    c. Trap oxygen so it remains in the airways
    d. Prevent the entrance of carbon dioxide into the airways

16. Which of the regions of the nose houses the conchae?
    a. Respiratory
    b. Vestibular
    c. Olfactory
    d. Medulla

17. Inert gas, in the context of the respiratory system, means:
    a. It is poisonous to the continuation of life
    b. It does not combine or interact in the body
    c. It is necessary for sustaining life
    d. It is depleting slowly from the atmosphere

18. The process of gas exchange in which carbon dioxide is removed from the blood and oxygen added is called:
    a. Internal respiration
    b. Internal ventilation
    c. External respiration
    d. External ventilation

19. Arrange the following gases from highest to lowest percent in the atmosphere.
    a. Oxygen, carbon dioxide, nitrogen, argon
    b. Nitrogen, oxygen, argon, carbon dioxide
    c. Oxygen, carbon dioxide, argon, nitrogen
    d. Carbon dioxide, hydrogen, oxygen, argon

20. The largest source of oxygen released into the atmosphere is from the:
    a. Ozone layer
    b. Fossil fuel
    c. Sahara desert
    d. Rain forest

21. Where does the upper airway or upper respiratory tract end?
    a. Just below the nasopharynx
    b. Just below the vocal cords
    c. Just below the trachea
    d. Just behind the nasal cavity

22. What is the principal function of the vestibular region of the nose?
    a. Filter out large particles
    b. Internal respiration
    c. Smell
    d. Phonation

23. The bulk movement of air down to the lungs is termed:
    a. Ventilation
    b. Respiration
    c. Transgasideous migration
    d. Pulmonary peristalsis

24. Where is the olfactory region of the nose?
    a. Behind the nostril to the sides of the cartilage
    b. Against the septum of the nasal cavity
    c. The rear of the nasal cavity on the tops of the uvula and soft palate
    d. Roof of the nasal cavity

25. Which of the following is not a function of the upper airway?
    a. Heating and cooling of inspired air
    b. Phonation
    c. Olfaction
    d. External respiration

MATCHING EXERCISES

Set 1

_____ 1. Rectus abdominis
_____ 2. External intercostals
_____ 3. Vibrissae
_____ 4. Vertebrocostal
_____ 5. Phrenic
_____ 6. Medulla oblongata
_____ 7. Turbinate
_____ 8. Vertebrosternal
_____ 9. Sternum
_____ 10. Carina

a. Receptors of smell
b. Conchae
c. Nose hair
d. True ribs
e. Breastbone
f. Nerve that innervates the diaphragm
g. Muscle of expiration
h. Respiratory control center
i. Muscle of inspiration
j. Where the trachea ends and primary bronchi begins
k. False ribs

Set 2

_____ 1. Capillary endothelium

_____ 2. Squamous pneumocytes

_____ 3. Terminal bronchiole

_____ 4. Alveolar epithelium

_____ 5. Interstitial

_____ 6. Pores of Kohn

_____ 7. Macrophages

_____ 8. Surfactant

_____ 9. Respiratory bronchioles

_____ 10. Granular pneumocytes

a. Coats the innermost layer of the alveoli

b. Marks the end of the conducting area of the lower respiratory tract

c. Leads to the alveolar ducts

d. Allows type III cells to move from one alveolus to another

e. Make up the majority of the actual tissue layer of the alveolus

f. Ingests foreign particles as they wander through the alveoli

g. Produce a phospholipid substance that acts on surface tension

h. Forms the walls of the blood vessels surrounding alveoli

i. Space that separates the alveoli from the capillaries

j. The actual tissue layer of the air sac functional units

k. Substance that increases surface tension

Set 3

_____ 1. Pneumonia

_____ 2. Tuberculosis

_____ 3. Emphysema

_____ 4. Hydrothorax

_____ 5. Erythropoietin

_____ 6. Asthma

_____ 7. Pneumothorax

_____ 8. Atelectasis

_____ 9. Hemoglobin

_____ 10. Hemothorax

a. Molecule that carries large amounts of oxygen

b. Constriction of the airway in response to an allergy

c. Clinical term for the influenza virus

d. Infectious disease; vast lung damage can occur

e. Lung infection; inflammation with accumulation of cell debris and fluid

f. Blood in the pleural space

g. When the air sacs of the lungs are partially or totally collapsed

h. Air in the thoracic cavity

i. Hormone that influences RBC production

j. Irreversible condition in which air sacs become destroyed

k. Fluid accumulation in the pleural space

FILL IN THE BLANK

1. When air is breathed into the body via the nose, it is moistened to _____ relative humidity.

2. The three sections of the pharynx are the _____, the _____, and the _____.

3. The voice box is clinically known as the _____.

4. The common name for the trachea is the _____.

5. Approximately _____ people die from smoking-related respiratory disease every year in the United States.

6. The region of the lung called the _____ is where pulmonary arteries exit, pulmonary veins enter, and the main stem of the bronchus can be found entering the lung.

7. The principal muscle of inspiration is called the _____.

8. The right lung has _____ lobes and the left lung has _____ lobes.

9. A substance called surfactant can be found in the _____.

10. Both men and women have _____ pairs of ribs, _____ of which are true ribs and _____ are floating ribs.

11. Located just above the clavicle is the _____ of the lungs.

12. When thoracic volume increases, the thoracic pressure _____.

13. The gas exchange surface of the lung is/are the _____.

14. When we exercise or participate in strenuous work, depth of breathing _____ and rate of breathing _____.

15. The eustachian tubes lead from the _____ to the _____.

SHORT ANSWER

1. Why is ridding the nose of its hair not advantageous?

_____

_____

_____

_____

2. What are the primary functions of the respiratory system?

_____

_____

_____

_____

3. Besides the diaphragm, what muscles play a role in inspiration? How do they aid inspiration?

_____

_____

_____

_____

4. Contrast internal and external respiration.

_____

_____

_____

_____

5. Explain why foreign objects are most likely to lodge in the right lung.

_____

_____

_____

_____

○ LABELING ACTIVITY

Label the various structures using Figure 13–1 on page 305 of your textbook as a guide.

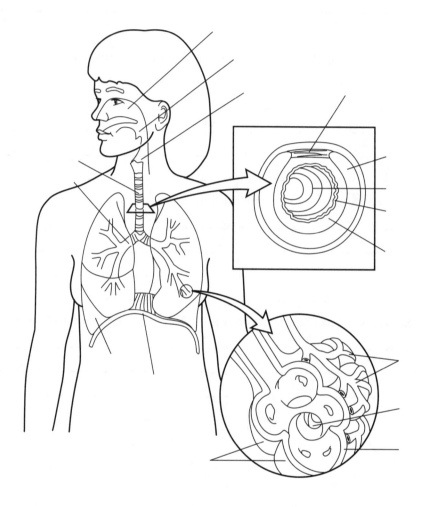

THE LYMPHATIC AND IMMUNE SYSTEMS: YOUR DEFENSE SYSTEMS

Chapter 14

MULTIPLE CHOICE

1. Which stage of cancer is often terminal?
    a. 4
    b. 3
    c. 2
    d. 1

2. Physical barriers of the immune system include:
    a. Skin
    b. Mucous membranes
    c. Saliva
    d. All of the above

3. How do antibodies destroy pathogens?
    a. May cause the antigens to clump
    b. Pinocytosis
    c. Phagocytosis
    d. Pull the antigen to the body surface, ulcerate the skin, and then release the antigen to the external environment

4. What do the lymphatic system, innate immunity, and adaptive immunity have in common?
    a. Rid the body of invading pathogens
    b. Lay dormant until needed
    c. Never turn on themselves
    d. Get stronger and better with age

5. After the physical barriers, which of the following is considered the first line of defense in the body?
    a. Antibodies
    b. Histamines
    c. Heparin
    d. Phagocytosis

6. The function of the spleen is to:
    a. Produce red blood cells
    b. Differentiate T lymphocytes
    c. Help WBCs mature
    d. Filter pathogens from the bloodstream

7. The right lymphatic duct empties into the:
   a. Thoracic duct
   b. Jugular vein
   c. Subclavian vein
   d. Spleen

8. How does lymph move through the body?
   a. Body movement
   b. Heart
   c. Gravity
   d. Centrifugal force

9. Lymphatic trunks empty into:
   a. Collecting ducts
   b. Subclavian veins
   c. Lymph nodes
   d. Thymus

10. Where is the spleen located?
    a. Between the heart and the sternum
    b. Upper right quadrant of abdomen
    c. Upper left quadrant of pelvis
    d. Upper left quadrant of abdomen

11. Which of the following areas have large concentrations of lymph nodes?
    a. Lumbar
    b. Subclavian
    c. Inguinal
    d. All of the above

12. Where do lymphocytes originate?
    a. Yellow bone marrow
    b. Red bone marrow
    c. Spleen
    d. Lymph nodes

13. Which one of the WBCs does the human immunodeficiency virus specifically target?
    a. Helper B cells
    b. Helper T cells
    c. Plasma cells
    d. Macrophages

14. Antibodies passed on to a fetus through the placenta represent:
    a. Innate immunity
    b. Naturally acquired passive immunity
    c. Artificially acquired passive immunity
    d. Naturally acquired active immunity

15. Lymph from the lower extremities will eventually empty into the:
    a. Femoral vein
    b. Inferior vena cava
    c. Right axillary vein
    d. None of the above

16. A vaccine is an example of:
    a. Innate immunity
    b. Artificially acquired active immunity
    c. Artificially acquired passive immunity
    d. Naturally acquired active immunity

17. Which of the following is/are lymphatic trunks?
    a. Axillary
    b. Jugular
    c. Cervical
    d. All of the above

18. Which of the following is true about the spleen?
    a. It is not a vital organ
    b. It produces red blood cells
    c. As we age, we rely on the spleen more
    d. All of the above are true

19. Which WBC is the first to arrive at the site of damage?
    a. Macrophage
    b. Plasma
    c. Neutrophils
    d. Lymphocytes

20. Biological increase in body temperature due to infection represents:
    a. Innate immunity
    b. Naturally acquired passive immunity
    c. Artificially acquired passive immunity
    d. Naturally acquired active immunity

21. Injection of antibiotics like penicillin is an example of:
    a. Naturally acquired active immunity
    b. Naturally acquired passive immunity
    c. Artificially acquired passive immunity
    d. None of the above

22. Which of the following vessels collects two thirds of the body's lymph?
    a. Inguinal duct
    b. Thoracic duct
    c. Right lymphatic duct
    d. Splenic duct

23. Which of the following WBCs are the most common in the bloodstream?
    a. Lymphocytes
    b. Monocytes
    c. Basophils
    d. Neutrophils

24. Where is the thymus located?
    a. Neck
    b. Chest
    c. Upper abdomen
    d. Brain

25. Which of the following is true about the function of the thymus gland?
    a. It has a higher functioning capacity in children than adults
    b. It contains lymphocytes
    c. It secretes a hormone
    d. All of the above

MATCHING EXERCISES

Set 1

_____ 1. Leukocyte

_____ 2. Neutrophil

_____ 3. Interferon

_____ 4. Macrophage

_____ 5. Basophil

_____ 6. Eosinophil

_____ 7. Natural killer cells

_____ 8. Dendritic cell

_____ 9. Cytotoxic

_____ 10. Plasma cells

a. Phagocytic granulocytes; most common WBC

b. Release chemicals to promote inflammation

c. All-encompassing term for white blood cells

d. Adaptive immunity T lymphocyte

e. Cytokine that protects neighboring cells from viral attack

f. Phagocytotic modified monocytes; innate immunity

g. Produces antibodies

h. Counteracts activity of basophils; active during parasitic infections

i. Modified monocytes acting as antigen-displaying cells

j. Innate lymphocytes that secrete chemicals to kill cells displaying antigens

Set 2

_____ 1. Primary immune response

_____ 2. Secondary immune response

_____ 3. Cell-mediated immunity

_____ 4. Turn-off immune response

_____ 5. Natural active immunity

_____ 6. Artificial passive immunity

_____ 7. Artificial active immunity

_____ 8. Natural passive immunity

_____ 9. Innate immunity

_____ 10. Tumor necrosis factor inhibitor

a. Memory B cells

b. Plasma cell

c. Perforin

d. Regulatory T cells

e. Treats rheumatoid arthritis

f. Physical barrier

g. The flu shot

h. Accidentally exposed to a pathogen like chicken pox

i. Being injected with antibodies

j. Breast milk

Set 3

_____ 1. Memory cells

_____ 2. Histamines

_____ 3. Interleukin-1

_____ 4. Lymph

_____ 5. Antigens

_____ 6. Fungi

_____ 7. Radiation

_____ 8. Venoms

_____ 9. Interleukin-2

_____ 10. Antibodies

a. Secreted by helper T cells

b. Located on cell surface

c. Remembers pathogens

d. Secreted by macrophages

e. Pathogenic organism

f. Inflammation-causing physical agent

g. Inflammation-causing chemical agent

h. Secreted by mast cells

i. Carries antigens to nodes around the body

j. Secreted by the plasma cells

FILL IN THE BLANK

1. When your body mounts a hyperactive response to a harmless antigen, the reaction is called a(n) _____.

2. The lymphatic tissue inside the lymph nodes contains _____ and _____.

3. The destruction of self-recognizing lymphocytes is known as

_____.

4. Helper T cells are also called _____ cells.

5. In order to fight off thousands of pathogens, lymphocytes must make thousands of copies of themselves. This process is called lymphocyte

_____.

6. A hypersensitivity reaction called _____ leads to _____ blood pressure and heart failure.

7. The thoracic duct empties into the _____.

8. The _____ produces a hormone that stimulates lymphocyte production in children.

9. When cancer has spread to nearby lymph nodes, it is in stage

_____.

10. The part of the brain that regulates body temperature is the

_____.

11. The lymphatic tissue inside a lymph node is surrounded by

_____.

12. During an allergic reaction, pollen directly activates the release of

_____.

13. Redness, swelling, heat, and possible pain are all _____ symptoms.

14. The formed elements in whole blood consist of erythrocytes, platelets, and _____.

15. Interferon and interleukins are both chemicals collectively called

_____.

SHORT ANSWER

1. Besides through viruses like the HIV that causes AIDS, how can a patient's immune system become compromised?

_____

_____

_____

_____

2. What is the primary function of lymph nodes?

_____

_____

_____

_____

3. Structurally contrast the spleen and large lymph nodes.

_____

_____

_____

_____

4. What is the purpose of a fever?

_____

_____

_____

_____

5. Why are CD-4 cells so important?

_____

_____

_____

_____

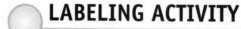

LABELING ACTIVITY

In the box provided, list the functions of each part of the lymphatic system and label the identified structures using Figure 4–14 on page 87 of your textbook as a guide.

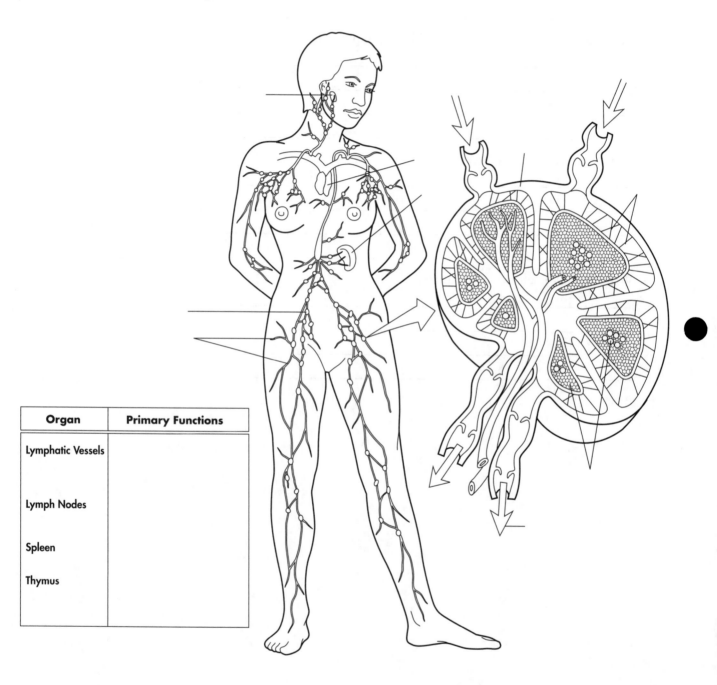

Organ	Primary Functions
Lymphatic Vessels	
Lymph Nodes	
Spleen	
Thymus	

THE GASTROINTESTINAL SYSTEM: FUEL FOR THE TRIP

Chapter 15

MULTIPLE CHOICE

1. Which of the salivary glands is found on the roof of the mouth?
   a. Parotid
   b. Submandibular
   c. Sublingual
   d. None of the above

2. If not pulled or knocked out, how many permanent teeth do we have by 25 years of age?
   a. 32
   b. 16
   c. 28
   d. 42

3. Please arrange the segments of the large intestine in the order waste travels through.
   a. Cecum, descending colon, ascending colon, transverse colon, sigmoid colon, rectum
   b. Cecum, ascending colon, transverse colon, descending colon, sigmoid colon, rectum
   c. Sigmoid colon, ascending colon, transverse colon, descending colon, cecum, rectum
   d. Sigmoid colon, descending colon, ascending colon, transverse colon, cecum, rectum

4. When food enters the mouth it is said to be:
   a. Ingested
   b. Digested
   c. Absorbed
   d. All of the above

5. The digestive enzyme secreted by the pancreas that when activated in the small intestine will digest proteins in food:
   a. Peptidase
   b. Amylase
   c. Pepsin
   d. Cholecystokinin

6. Where does 80 percent of absorption of usable nutrients take place?
   a. Stomach
   b. Mouth
   c. Large intestine
   d. Small intestine

7. Which nerve innervates the visceral muscles of the stomach causing contraction and hence motility?
   a. Phrenic
   b. Vagus
   c. Trigeminal
   d. Sciatic

8. The *labia* is/are commonly known as the:
   a. Tongue
   b. Gallbladder
   c. Lips
   d. Uvula

9. What does *emulsify* mean in terms of fat?
   a. The building of fatty acid chains in the liver
   b. The binding of fatty acids to carrier proteins for transport to the liver
   c. The destruction of fat globules or the rendering of fat globules unusable so no absorption will ever take place
   d. The breaking down or converting of fat into a form that promotes enzymatic chemical digestion

10. Which sphincter lies between the stomach and small intestine?
    a. Cardiac
    b. Gastroenteral
    c. Pyloric
    d. Ileocecal

11. What is the pH (acidity) of HCl in the stomach?
    a. 1.5 to 2.0
    b. 7.0 to 7.2
    c. 7.5 to 8.8
    d. 12.0 to 13.6

12. What is the function of the liver?
    a. Detoxify
    b. Produce clotting factors
    c. Store glucose in a form called glycogen
    d. All of the above

13. What is a *lacteal*, and where is it located?
    a. Lymphatic capillary in each villus of small intestine
    b. Blood capillary beside goblet cells in the pancreas
    c. Enzyme in the pancreas that, when secreted, digests milk
    d. Mucous lining found in the stomach

14. In the stomach, what do the parietal cells secrete, and what do the chief cells secrete?
    a. Sucrose/fructose
    b. Amylase/lipase

c. HCl/pepsinogen

    d. Bile/bilirubin

15. In reference to the cardiac sphincter, where is the fundus of the stomach?

    a. Left, superior

    b. Right, inferior

    c. Left, inferior

    d. Right, superior

16. What structure prevents us from swallowing our tongue and also aids in proper speaking?

    a. Diaphragm

    b. Uvula

    c. Epiglottis

    d. Frenulum

17. Which section of the small intestine connects to or is continuous with the stomach?

    a. Cecum

    b. Duodenum

    c. Ileum

    d. Jejunum

18. Which of the following statements is correct?

    a. The hepatic ducts conduct bile from the liver, the cystic duct conducts bile to and from the gallbladder, and the common bile duct conducts bile to the small intestine

    b. The common bile duct conducts bile from the liver, the cystic duct conducts bile to and from the gallbladder, and the hepatic ducts conduct bile to the small intestine

    c. The cystic duct conducts bile from the liver, the hepatic ducts conduct bile to and from the gallbladder, and the common bile duct conducts bile to the small intestine

    d. The common bile duct conducts bile from the liver, the hepatic ducts conduct bile to and from the gallbladder, and the cystic ducts conduct bile to the small intestine

19. Where is the most common region for peptic ulcer disease?

    a. Distal and middle parts of the esophagus

    b. Body of the stomach

    c. Upper or proximal part of small intestine

    d. Rectum and around the anal sphincter

20. The vermiform appendix hangs off the:

    a. Cecum

    b. Rectum

    c. Colon

    d. Ileum

21. What effect does secretin have on the stomach?

    a. Increases muscular activity

    b. Produces bile

    c. Increases secretions

    d. Decreases overall activity

22. How many incisors do adults normally have?
    a. 4
    b. 6
    c. 8
    d. 10

23. The uvula is associated with which structure?
    a. Soft palate
    b. Hard palate
    c. Tongue
    d. Pharynx

24. What substance starts chemically breaking down in the mouth due to salivary secretions?
    a. Starch
    b. Protein
    c. Fat
    d. Lactose

25. Bilirubin from what is eliminated in bile?
    a. Fat
    b. Food
    c. Feces
    d. Blood cells

MATCHING EXERCISES

Set 1

_____ 1. Cirrhosis
_____ 2. Enteritis
_____ 3. Anorexia
_____ 4. Calculi
_____ 5. Hemorrhoids
_____ 6. Crohn's disease
_____ 7. Gingivitis
_____ 8. Gastritis
_____ 9. Bulimia
_____ 10. Cholecystitis

a. Disease marked with "binge-purge" of food
b. Inflammation of the stomach
c. Chronic disease of the liver
d. Inflammation of the gallbladder
e. Constipation or fecal impacting at the transverse colon
f. Regional ileitis
g. Inflammation of the small intestine
h. Disease marked by loss of appetite and remarkable weight loss
i. Inflammation of the gums
j. Varicose veins of the rectum
k. Gallstones

Set 2

_____ 1. Secretin
_____ 2. Cholecystokinin
_____ 3. Pepsin
_____ 4. Hydrochloric acid
_____ 5. Bile
_____ 6. Peptidase
_____ 7. Intrinsic factor
_____ 8. Gastrin
_____ 9. Sucrase
_____ 10. Amylase

a. Breaks down protein in stomach
b. Emulsifies fat
c. Breaks down starches in mouth
d. Neutralizes the chyme in duodenum
e. Needed for the absorption of B_{12}
f. Stimulates the release of bile
g. Breaks down disaccharides
h. Breaks down protein in small intestines
i. Hormone that increases gastric activity
j. Digests portions of protein structures in small intestine
k. Converts pepsinogen to pepsin
l. Hormone that activates bile production

Set 3

_____ 1. Chyle
_____ 2. Rugae
_____ 3. Gingiva
_____ 4. Peyer's patch
_____ 5. Adventitia
_____ 6. Villi
_____ 7. Epiglottis
_____ 8. Nitroglycerine
_____ 9. Cementum
_____ 10. Bolus

a. Medication used to increase gastric juices
b. Folds in the stomach
c. Anchors root of tooth to gums
d. Lymph tissue in small intestine
e. Food stuff mixed with salivary juices
f. Food stuff mixed with gastric juices
g. Fingerlike protrusions in small intestine
h. Absorbable under the tongue
i. Gum
j. Serosa of the esophagus
k. Prevents food from slipping into lungs
l. Lipoproteins in the lacteal formed from glycerol and fatty acids

FILL IN THE BLANK

1. Any organ the function and size of which seem to have been reduced as humans evolved is termed _____.

2. Another name for canine teeth is _____.

3. Gastric activities, such as churning and secretion of enzymes, are controlled by the _____ nervous system (be specific).

4. For most of the digestive tract, the serosa layer is also called _____.

5. Between the ages of 2 and 3, all _____ of your baby teeth should have appeared.

6. The clinical term for the elimination of unusable material from the body is _____.

7. The digestive tract is also called the _____ tract.

8. If fecal material moves through the large intestine too fast, _____ occurs.

9. Now violently coughing, client A was previously eating and talking at the same time. Her partially chewed beef jerky slipped by her _____, which closes off her airway when she swallows.

10. The three main regions of the large intestine are the _____, _____, and _____.

11. Besides food from the stomach, the first part of the small intestine receives additional secretions from the _____ and the _____.

12. Baby teeth are clinically called _____ teeth.

13. Heartburn occurs when the _____ opens and there is a backflow of food.

14. The digestive enzyme found in saliva is _____.

15. If fecal material moves too slowly through the intestine, _____ occurs.

SHORT ANSWER

1. What is the purpose of villi, plicae circularis, and microvilli in the small intestine?

_____

_____

_____

_____

2. Why do lactose-intolerant people suffer from diarrhea and bloating if they consume milk or milk products?

_____

_____

_____

_____

3. Although it produces powerful enzymes and chemicals, why doesn't the stomach digest itself?

_____

_____

_____

_____

4. List and describe the location of the three named salivary glands.

_____

_____

_____

_____

5. What is the importance of digestion?

_____

_____

_____

_____

120 Chapter 15

LABELING ACTIVITY

Draw a line from the organ label to the correct organ on the figure. Color code each structure using Figure 4–15 on page 88 of your textbook as a guide.

Organ	Primary Functions
Salivary Glands	Provide lubrication, produce buffers and the enzymes that begin digestion
Pharynx	Passageway connected to esophagus
Esophagus	Delivers food to stomach
Stomach	Secretes acids and enzymes
Small Intestine	Secretes digestive enzymes, absorbs nutrients
Liver	Secretes bile, regulates blood composition of nutrients
Gallbladder	Stores bile for release into small intestine
Pancreas	Secretes digestive enzymes and buffers; contains endocrine cells
Large Intestine	Removes water from fecal material, stores waste

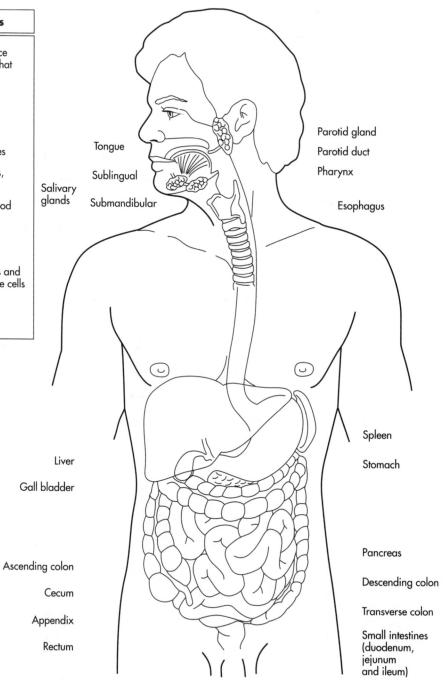

Tongue

Sublingual

Salivary glands

Submandibular

Parotid gland

Parotid duct

Pharynx

Esophagus

Spleen

Stomach

Liver

Gall bladder

Pancreas

Descending colon

Transverse colon

Ascending colon

Cecum

Appendix

Rectum

Small intestines (duodenum, jejunum and ileum)

THE URINARY SYSTEM: FILTRATION AND FLUID BALANCE

Chapter 16

MULTIPLE CHOICE

1. The renal capsule covers the:
   a. Kidney
   b. Glomerulus
   c. Bladder
   d. Afferent arteriole

2. Which of the following will not pass through the glomerular epithelium into the nephron?
   a. RBC
   b. WBC
   c. Protein molecules
   d. All of the above

3. Compared to the concentration in urine, in glomerular filtrate, glucose is:
   a. At the same concentration
   b. At a higher concentration
   c. At a lower concentration
   d. None of the above

4. The urinary bladder walls are composed of what type of muscle?
   a. Smooth
   b. Voluntary
   c. Skeletal
   d. b and c

5. One of the symptoms of kidney stones:
   a. Pale urine
   b. Blood in urine
   c. Lower back numbness
   d. Excessive, uncontrollable, painless urination with continual expulsion of crystalline structures

6. Compared to the concentration in urine, in plasma, urea is:
   a. At the same concentration
   b. At a higher concentration
   c. At a lower concentration
   d. None of the above

7. Besides water, which of the following substances is usually found in urine at the bladder level?
   a. Glucose
   b. Ammonia
   c. Amino acids
   d. All of the above

8. Where are the kidneys located?
   a. Upper abdomen
   b. Lower abdomen
   c. Scrotal sac
   d. Pelvic cavity

9. Which of the urinary organs transports urine from the kidneys to the bladder?
   a. Nephrons
   b. Urethras
   c. Ureters
   d. Glomerulus

10. Compared to glomerular filtrate, in urine, urea and creatinine are:
    a. At the same concentration
    b. At a higher concentration
    c. At a lower concentration
    d. None of the above

11. Compared to urine, in plasma, sodium is:
    a. At the same concentration
    b. At a higher concentration
    c. At a lower concentration
    d. None of the above

12. In which layer of the kidney is blood filtered?
    a. Pelvis
    b. Medulla
    c. Cortex
    d. Capsule

13. Which of the following structures is located in the renal medulla?
    a. Major calyces
    b. Pyramids
    c. Glomerulus
    d. Minor calyces

14. Normally, how can we consciously control the expulsion of urine from the body?
    a. Conscious control over the urinary bladder muscle
    b. Conscious control over the ureter sphincters
    c. Conscious control over the urethral sphincters
    d. Conscious control over the production of urine

15. Which of the following is the correct order in which blood arrives at the glomerulus?
    a. Renal artery, peritubular, arcuate, lobular, lobar, segmental, efferent arteriole

b. Renal artery, arcuate, segmental, lobar, lobular, interlobular, afferent arteriole

c. Renal artery, lobar, interlobar, lobular, interlobular, arcuate, efferent arteriole

d. Renal artery, segmental, lobar, interlobar, arcuate, interlobular, afferent arteriole

16. Blood leaves the kidney's hilum via the:
    a. Renal artery
    b. Inferior vena cava
    c. Efferent arteriole
    d. Renal vein

17. As blood travels through the vessels that surround the nephrons, it exits the kidneys through a series of vessels that are in direct reverse of the arteries with one exception:
    a. There are no arcuate veins
    b. There are no segmental veins
    c. There are no lobular or lobar veins
    d. There are extra veins called the juxtaglomedullary veins

18. Compared to glomerular filtrate, in plasma, sodium and potassium are:
    a. At the same concentration
    b. At a higher concentration
    c. At a lower concentration
    d. None of the above

19. What happens at the Bowman's capsule?
    a. Excretion
    b. Secretion
    c. Filtration
    d. Reabsorption

20. Which of the following usually makes up a sizable portion of glomerular filtrate?
    a. Red blood cells and proteins
    b. White blood cells and proteins
    c. Water and glucose
    d. Ammonia and hydrogen ions

21. Which of the following is secreted at the nephron?
    a. Red blood cells and proteins
    b. White blood cells and sodium
    c. Water and glucose
    d. Ammonia and hydrogen ions

22. Glomerular filtrate flows from the renal corpuscle into the:
    a. Loop of Henle
    b. Proximal convoluted tubules
    c. Distal convoluted tubules
    d. Collecting ducts

23. Which of the following is either completely or partially reabsorbed, respectively, at the nephron?
    a. Red blood cells and potassium
    b. White blood cells and proteins
    c. Glucose and water
    d. Ammonia and hydrogen ions

24. Glomerular filtrate flows from the distal convoluted tubules into the:
    a. Collecting ducts
    b. Ascending limb of the loop of Henle
    c. Descending limb of the loop of Henle
    d. Proximal convoluted tubules

25. When systemic blood pressure has increased, what protective measures do the kidneys take?
    a. Vasodilate
    b. Vasoconstrict
    c. Shut down one kidney
    d. Nephrotic necrosis (spontaneous death of the nephrons)

MATCHING EXERCISES

Set 1

_____ 1. PKD

_____ 2. Analgesic nephropathy

_____ 3. Diabetes insipidus

_____ 4. Diabetes mellitus

_____ 5. Water toxicity

_____ 6. Glomerulosclerosis

_____ 7. Hemolytic uremic syndrome

_____ 8. Kidney stones

_____ 9. Hematuria

_____ 10. Urinary tract infection

a. Dangerously low blood sodium

b. Nephrons are replaced by cysts

c. Means blood in the urine

d. Movement of fecal matter into urethra and bladder

e. Scarring of portions of the renal corpuscles

f. May be caused by overuse of ibuprofen

g. Insulin deficiency and hyperglycemia

h. RBC debris may block vessels to kidney

i. Too little antidiuretic hormone being produced and secreted

j. Can block kidney tubules

Set 2

_____ 1. Rugae
_____ 2. Diffusion
_____ 3. Osmosis
_____ 4. Voiding
_____ 5. Filtration
_____ 6. Secretion
_____ 7. Reabsorption
_____ 8. Autoregulation
_____ 9. Vasoconstriction
_____ 10. Vasodilation

a. Increase of blood vessel diameter

b. Decrease of blood vessel diameter

c. Movement of ions and solutes from high to low concentration

d. Urination

e. Permits expansion of the urinary bladder

f. Movement of substances from tubules to capillaries

g. Controls blood pressure to nephrons

h. Movement of water from low ion to high ion concentration

i. Movement of blood substances from glomerulus into capsule

j. Movement of substances from capillaries to tubules

Set 3

_____ 1. Ureter
_____ 2. Urethra
_____ 3. Kidney
_____ 4. Bladder
_____ 5. Nephron
_____ 6. Renal hilum
_____ 7. Renal pyramid
_____ 8. Minor calyces
_____ 9. Juxtaglomerular
_____ 10. Peritubular capillaries

a. Bean-shaped structure that filters blood and forms urine

b. Functional unit of the kidney

c. Striped areas in the renal medulla; collection of renal tubules

d. Transports urine from kidneys to bladder

e. Transports urine to outside the body

f. Wraps around nephrons; participates in secretion and reabsorption

g. Indentation on medial side of kidneys

h. Monitors blood flow to kidneys; secretes renin

i. Receives filtrate from collecting duct

j. Hollow holding structure for urine

FILL IN THE BLANK

1. The three processes necessary to clean blood and make urine are

   _____, _____, and

   _____.

2. The vessels called _____ bring blood to the

   glomerulus, and the vessels called _____ leave the

   glomerulus with the unfiltered blood components.

3. The nephron is divided into two distinct parts called the

   _____ and the _____.

4. Beverages such as _____ and _____

   inhibit ADH secretion.

5. The noninvasive treatment to break up kidney stones, called

   _____, involves shock waves.

6. The leading cause of kidney failure in the United States is

   _____.

7. The hormone that acts to retain more sodium in the body is

   _____.

8. High blood and urine glucose (sugar) is characteristic of a disorder called

   _____.

9. The three structures found at the renal hilum are the

   _____, _____, and

   _____.

10. The innermost region or layer of the kidney is the

    _____.

11. The functional unit of the kidney is the _____.

12. Glomerular filtrate flows from the proximal convoluted tubules into the

    _____.

13. When molecules move from the capillary network into the distal

    convoluted tubules, that movement is termed _____.

14. The substances that are not filtered through the glomerular epithelium

    into the renal corpuscle and tubules are directed into the

    _____ vessels.

15. Contraction of the urinary bladder muscles is controlled by

    _____ neurons of the autonomic nervous system.

SHORT ANSWER

1. Why are urinary tract infections more common in women than in men?

_____

_____

_____

_____

2. In maintaining homeostasis and in reference to the urinary system, how does autoregulation work?

_____

_____

_____

_____

3. How does the body regulate pH if too much acid is present in the blood?

_____

_____

_____

_____

4. In what way are aldosterone and atrial natriuretic hormones antagonists?

_____

_____

_____

_____

5. Why would a person who survives a trauma resulting in massive blood loss fall victim to kidney damage or permanent renal failure?

_____

_____

_____

_____

LABELING ACTIVITY

List the organs that correspond to the functions listed in the box and label the illustrations using Figure 4–16 on page 89 of your textbook as a guide.

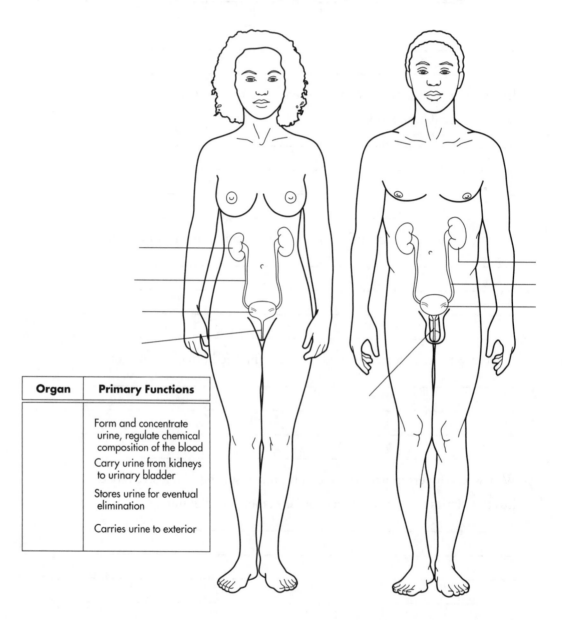

Organ	Primary Functions
	Form and concentrate urine, regulate chemical composition of the blood
	Carry urine from kidneys to urinary bladder
	Stores urine for eventual elimination
	Carries urine to exterior

THE REPRODUCTIVE SYSTEM: REPLACEMENT AND REPAIR

Chapter 17

MULTIPLE CHOICE

1. The external opening of the vagina may be covered by a perforated membrane called the:
   a. Prepuce
   b. Foreskin
   c. Hymen
   d. Fimbria

2. BPH is a pathology marked by:
   a. Breast polyps commonly seen in women over 50
   b. Biological pelvic heliobacterium that affects prepuberty girls
   c. Prostate enlargement commonly seen in males over 50
   d. Hermaphroditic pelvic organs caused by fetal hormone imbalance

3. In patients with erectile dysfunction disorder:
   a. The penis lacks blood vessels in the shafts
   b. The penis in unable to lose an erection
   c. Men are unable to make viable sperm
   d. The penis is not able to have a full erection

4. Uterine tubes are *not*:
   a. The birth canal
   b. The oviducts
   c. The fallopian tubes
   d. Where fertilization takes place

5. How many chromosomes does a zygote have in each cell?
   a. 42
   b. 46
   b. 21
   d. 16 pairs

6. The primary male genitalia is/are the:
   a. Penis
   b. Testicles
   c. Sperm
   d. Muscles

7. Which of the following are part of the spermatic cord?
   a. Vas deferens, ejaculatory duct, epididymis
   b. Testes, vas deferens, nerves
   c. Vas deferens, nerves, blood vessels
   d. Blood vessels, ejaculatory duct, penis

8. In most cases, vaginitis is caused by:
   a. Microorganisms
   b. Macroorganisms
   c. Radiation
   d. Trauma

9. In a pap smear, scrapings from what area are examined for precancerous cells?
   a. Cervix
   b. Vaginal walls
   c. Uterine walls
   d. Ovarian surface

10. Hydrocele is an abnormal collection of fluid in the:
    a. Ovaries
    b. Breasts
    c. Testes
    d. Uterus

11. What may cause amenorrhea?
    a. Emotional distress
    b. Extreme dieting
    c. Poor health
    d. All of the above

12. When a vasectomy is performed, what is prevented from traveling out of the penis during intercourse?
    a. semen
    b. testosterone
    c. sperm
    d. urine

13. An IUD is:
    a. A contractible disease: inflammatory urethral disease
    b. A means of contraception
    c. A means of conception
    d. Gamete deformity

14. When the loose skin covering the tip of the penis is removed, whether in infancy or adulthood, the male is then referred to as being:
    a. Circumcised
    b. Impotent
    c. Aroused
    d. Neutered

15. At what point is the developing human referred to as a fetus?
    a. At fertilization
    b. The eight-cell stage after fertilization
    c. At implantation
    d. Eight weeks after fertilization until birth

16. How many sperm can fertilize the egg?
    a. 2
    b. 1
    c. 42
    d. 23 pairs

17. The fetus floats in a fluid called:
    a. Amniotic
    b. Vestibular
    c. Semen
    d. Embryonic

18. Approximately at what age does sperm production end?
    a. 45
    b. 55
    c. 65
    d. Death

19. Where is the prostate gland located?
    a. In the glans penis
    b. In the scrotum
    c. Under the urinary bladder
    d. Lateral to the cervix

20. Which of the following layers of the uterus sheds when a woman has her period?
    a. Myometrium
    b. Perimetrium
    c. Functional layer of the mucosa
    d. Basal layer of the endometrium

21. The process of sorting chromosomes so that each gamete (egg or sperm) gets the right number of copies of the genetic material:
    a. Meiosis
    b. Fertilization
    c. Reduction division
    d. Mitosis

22. A surgeon wants to treat a tumor in the myometrium by occluding the arteries that serve that layer, without affecting the endometrium, perimetrium, or other pelvic structures. She will then attempt to occlude which arteries?
    a. Arcuate arteries
    b. Common iliac arteries
    c. Straight radial arteries
    d. Spiral radial arteries

23. Which structure of the female anatomy has great similarity to the penis in that it becomes engorged with blood during sexual arousal?
    a. Breast
    b. Ovaries
    c. Mons pubis
    d. Clitoris

24. What kind of feedback on the hypothalamus do estrogen and testosterone respectively exert?
    a. Negative/negative
    b. Negative/positive
    c. Positive/positive
    d. Positive/negative

25. Where does sperm mature?
    a. Epididymis
    b. Prostate
    c. Sertoli
    d. Penile shaft

MATCHING EXERCISES

Set 1

_____ 1. Cryptorchidism

_____ 2. Mastectomy

_____ 3. Vasectomy

_____ 4. Mastitis

_____ 5. Ectopic pregnancy

_____ 6. Abruptio placentae

_____ 7. Vaginitis

_____ 8. Breech

_____ 9. Dysmenorrhea

_____ 10. Amenorrhea

a. The placenta tears away from the uterine walls

b. Fertilized egg implants in fallopian tubes

c. Absence of menstruation

d. When the testes do not descend during late fetal development

e. Severing or tying off the vas deferens; a form of birth control

f. Inflammation of the breast tissue

g. Inflammation of the vagina

h. Fetus coming through the birth canal buttocks first

i. Difficult menstruation

j. Removal of breast usually because of cancer or debilitating tumors

Set 2

_____ 1. Gonads

_____ 2. Areola

_____ 3. Granulosa

_____ 4. Vestibule

_____ 5. Fimbria

_____ 6. Corpus albicans

_____ 7. Sertoli

_____ 8. Tunica vaginalis

_____ 9. Inguinal

_____ 10. Tunica albuginea

a. Space between labia minora where the urethra and vagina empty

b. Most superficial layer of connective tissue surrounding testes

c. General term for both the ovaries and testes

d. Fibrous capsule covering the ovaries

e. Canal where the vas deferens passes from scrotum to trunk

f. Helper cells for the sperm

g. Nipple

h. Helper cells surrounding the primary oocyte

i. Ciliated projection on the distal portion of both uterine tubes

j. A degenerating structure in the ovaries

Set 3

_____ 1. Semen

_____ 2. Prolactin

_____ 3. Oxytocin

_____ 4. Testosterone

_____ 5. Progesterone

_____ 6. Estrogen

_____ 7. Gonadotropin-releasing hormone

_____ 8. Follicle-stimulating hormone

_____ 9. Luteinizing hormone

_____ 10. Human chorionic gonadotropin

a. Rising levels stimulate proliferation of the uterine lining

b. Rising levels maintain the buildup of the endometrium

c. Hormone responsible for maintaining the corpus luteum

d. Substance containing sperm, mucus, sugars, and certain chemicals

e. Hormone-regulating contraction of uterus and ejection of milk

f. Responsible for masculinization at puberty

g. Regulates production and secretion of certain pituitary hormones

h. Initiates the development of primary follicle

i. In females, a surge in this hormone is coupled with ovulation

j. Hormone regulating the production of milk

FILL IN THE BLANK

1. The typical genetic makeup of humans is that females have the sex chromosomes _____ and males have _____.

2. The urethra in males transports both _____ and _____.

3. The production of sperm is termed _____.

4. A(n) _____ refers to the expansion of the penis upon sexual arousal.

5. Milk-secreting sacs in the mammary lobules are called _____.

6. Between the two halves of the labia majora is an opening known as the _____ cleft.

7. The secretory phase of menstruation is also known as the _____ phase.

8. Sperm, in one of the many ducts, pass by the _____ just before flowing into the ejaculatory duct.

9. A primary oocyte has _____ chromosomes.

10. In males, luteinizing and follicle-stimulating hormones are produced and secreted by the _____.

11. If not surgically removed, the loose tissue called _____ normally covers the tip of the penis.

12. The isthmus of the uterine tubes are connected to the _____ of the uterus.

13. The primary male genitalia is/are the _____.

14. In humans, testosterone is first secreted _____.

15. The valvelike structure of the uterus called the _____ protrudes into the vagina, and its characteristic dilation marks a certain stage in delivery.

SHORT ANSWER

1. Contrast the terms *menopause* and *menarche*.

   _____
   _____
   _____
   _____

2. Describe the three stages of labor.

   _____
   _____
   _____
   _____

3. Contrast the effect estrogen and progesterone have on the endometrium.

   _____
   _____
   _____
   _____

4. What determines the sex of a baby?

   _____
   _____
   _____
   _____

5. Trace the events of ejaculation from the scrotal sac to the release of semen into the vagina.

   _____
   _____
   _____
   _____

● LABELING ACTIVITY

Label the parts of the male and female reproductive system and identify the organs described in the Function Boxes using Figure 4–17 on page 90 of your textbook as a guide.

Organ	Primary Functions (female)
	Produce ova (eggs) and hormones
	Deliver ova or embryo to uterus; normal site of fertilization
	Site of development of offspring
	Site of sperm deposition; birth canal at delivery; provides passage of fluids during menstruation
	Erectile organ, produces pleasurable sensations during sexual act
	Contain glands that lubricate entrance to vagina
	Produce milk that nourishes newborn infant

Organ	Primary Functions (male)
	Produce sperm and hormones
	Site of sperm maturation
	Conducts sperm between epididymis and prostate
	Secrete fluid that makes up much of the volume of semen
	Secretes buffers and fluid
	Conducts semen to exterior
	Erectile organ used to deposit sperm in the vagina of a female; produces pleasurable sensations during sexual act
	Surrounds and positions the testes

THE JOURNEY'S END: NOW WHAT?

Chapter 18

MULTIPLE CHOICE

1. Bone scouring is an indication of:
   a. Tuberculosis
   b. Hepatitis
   c. Calcium deficiency
   d. High-impact mechanical stress

2. Which nerve is damaged in carpal tunnel syndrome?
   a. Median
   b. Acoustic
   c. Sciatic
   d. Radial

3. What bone fragment, showing evidence of primitive surgery, was found in a 400-year-old trash dump?
   a. Skull
   b. Femur
   c. Rib
   d. Sacrum

4. Who was Josef Mengele?
   a. The Merciless Hooded Ghost responsible for the brutality against Native Americans between 1812 and 1831
   b. The Fearless Ace responsible for "downing" several Allied Force fighter jets
   c. The Consignor of Hotel Hanoi responsible for the torture of many prisoners of war during the Vietnam War
   d. The Angel of Death responsible for the deaths of many humans during World War II

5. According to your text, what substance containing thallium was intentionally and secretly fed to the victim, causing his death.
   a. Rat poison
   b. Drain cleaner
   c. Paint thinner
   d. Motor oil

6. Which of the following is true about fingerprints?
   a. Only identical twins have the same fingerprints
   b. They are friction ridges on the hands and feet
   c. They are only fully formed between the first and second year of life
   d. All of the above

7. DNA fingerprinting helped determine that Thomas Jefferson, the third president of the United States, or a relative:
   a. Murdered his first wife
   b. Burglarized the White House repeatedly
   c. Fathered children of his slave
   d. Had Alzheimer's disease

8. In the elderly, what changes are seen in the taste buds?
   a. The acuity of salt becomes more sensitive
   b. The number of taste buds increases
   c. Sweet tastes become less discernable than bitter tastes
   d. All of the above

9. Although bone loss occurs in both men and women, the highest percentage bone loss in women can be seen:
   a. 10 years after menopause
   b. In the first 5 years postmenopause
   c. 6 months prior to menopause
   d. after age 70

10. As we age:
    a. Heart valves become soft
    b. Cardiac output decreases
    c. Blood pressure decreases
    d. All of the above

11. What is bone scouring?
    a. The thinning of the bone's cortex as a result of poor nutrition
    b. The thickening and extension of the trabeculae as a result of weight-bearing activities
    c. The malrepair of bones as a result of improper splinting or casting of a fractured bone
    d. The destruction of smooth bone surfaces as a result of colonization of bacteria

12. In forensic science, which anatomical structure is examined for evidence of tuberculosis?
    a. The skin
    b. The nasal apertures
    c. The retina of the left eye
    d. Ends of long bones

13. In the elderly, changes in the integumentary system include:
    a. Increased skin delicacy
    b. Loss of elasticity
    c. Multiple lesions
    d. All of the above

14. Stress:
    a. Is not a natural part of life and must be controlled
    b. Gives a false sense of security and protection
    c. Is good and necessary, but chronic stress may be problematic
    d. All of the above

15. Beneficial in maintaining healthy bones, what is recommended?
    a. Calcium and vitamins
    b. Weight-bearing exercises
    c. Repetitive motion such as typing
    d. a and b

16. What may cause carpal tunnel syndrome?
    a. Bright lights and abuse of such drugs as ecstasy
    b. Weight-bearing exercises
    c. Loud sounds and high pitches
    d. Repetitive motion such as playing the piano

17. For optimum health, how much water is recommended per day?
    a. 3 glasses
    b. 8 glasses
    c. 14 glasses
    d. 1 cup

18. What technique was initially used to confirm that Wolfgang Gerhard was really Josef Mengele?
    a. Video skull–face superimposition
    b. Fingerprints
    c. Voice recognition
    d. Reverse psychology and multiple interviews

19. Which of the following has/have an adverse effect on the cardiovascular system?
    a. Alcohol
    b. Smoking
    c. Saturated fats
    d. All of the above

20. Why can high doses of vitamin A, D, E, and K actually harm the body?
    a. Being water soluble, they tax the kidneys
    b. They deteriorate the stomach's lining
    c. They can build up to a toxic level
    d. They prevent absorption of proteins and carbohydrates

21. What is needed in order to identify a criminal suspect through DNA fingerprinting?
    a. Both blood and reproductive fluid from a crime scene
    b. Both DNA from a crime scene and a known DNA sample
    c. Both DNA from the mother and father of the accused
    d. Only the DNA from the crime scene

22. The simplest and most effective way to stop the spread of infections:
    a. Avoid contact
    b. Wash hands
    c. Drink more water
    d. Take antibiotics

23. An antibiotic cream or tablet is what kind of agent?
    a. Antifungal
    b. Antiviral
    c. Antiprotozoan
    d. Antibacterial

24. Which of the following is/are considered diuretics?
    a. Water
    b. Caffeinated coffee
    c. Gatorade
    d. a and c

25. The ability to roll your tongue is:
    a. Gender-specific
    b. Learned
    c. An inherited trait
    d. Race-specific

MATCHING EXERCISES

Set 1

_____   1. Vitamin A
_____   2. Calcium
_____   3. Vitamin B_1
_____   4. Vitamin B_{12}
_____   5. Vitamin C
_____   6. Niacin
_____   7. Vitamin E
_____   8. Vitamin K
_____   9. Vitamin D
_____ 10. Folic acid

a. Aids in the absorption of calcium from the gut

b. Facilitates fat synthesis and glycolysis

c. Recommended for proper night vision

d. Raw material for bones and teeth

e. Needed for hemolytic resistance of RBCs

f. Need to prevent spina bifida

g. Needed for carbohydrate metabolism and normal digestion and appetite

h. To treat pernicious anemia

i. Needed for proper blood clotting

j. Aids in the absorption of iron

Set 2

_____ 1. SIDS
_____ 2. Black lung
_____ 3. Lead poisoning
_____ 4. Genital warts
_____ 5. Syphilis
_____ 6. Herpes
_____ 7. Gonorrhea
_____ 8. Chlamydia
_____ 9. Melanoma
_____ 10. Tuberculosis

a. Common among coalminers
b. Human papilloma virus
c. Presents with fluid-filled vesicles on the genitalia
d. Presents with swollen testes and inflamed cervix
e. Skin cancer
f. Normally thought of as a bacterial pulmonary disease
g. Associated with infants
h. From pewter plates
i. Presents with degeneration of the nervous system
j. Presents with purulent discharge and abnormal menstruation

Set 3

Match the following systems with their appropriate age-related and/or wellness concerns.

_____ 1. Reproductive system
_____ 2. Immune system
_____ 3. Sensory system
_____ 4. Endocrine system
_____ 5. Brain and nervous system
_____ 6. Respiratory system
_____ 7. Skeletal system
_____ 8. Integumentary system
_____ 9. Cardiovascular system
_____ 10. Urinary system

a. Incontinence
b. Pain and stress
c. Clogged vessels
d. Antibiotics abuse
e. Smoking and emphysema
f. High level of noise
g. Steroid abuse
h. Skin cancer
i. Carpal tunnel syndrome
j. Smoking and SIDS

FILL IN THE BLANK

1. Ancient _____ were stricken with tuberculosis, as investigators discovered by examining their bones.

2. According to the text, a bone fragment indicative of primitive surgery was found in a 400-year-old trash dump in _____.

3. Administering many drugs at the same time is termed

_____.

4. In the absence of disease, the brain continues to mature up to the age of

_____.

5. Bone density usually reaches its greatest peak at _____.

6. In general, as an individual ages, he or she loses _____

and _____ and gains _____.

7. A pap smear is a test for cancer of the _____.

8. Anabolic steroids are closely related to the hormone

_____.

9. A mammogram is a test for cancer of the _____.

10. Approximately _____ people die annually in the

United States because of smoking-related disease.

11. The cancer treatment that uses energy waves rather than chemicals to

shrink tumors is called _____ therapy.

12. Clients who have the procedure called _____ done

usually were 26 percent less likely to have their cancer return within 5

years than clients who only had the tumor removed.

13. Smoking can lead to chronic respiratory diseases such as

_____, _____, and

_____.

14. CIPA is the acronym for _____.

15. According to your text, thallium was found in the victim's

_____, which linked the wife to the murder.

SHORT ANSWER

1. How does the sexually transmitted disease HPV present itself in both

males and females?

_____

_____

_____

_____

2. Besides completely staying out of the sun, in what ways can we prevent excessive sun exposure?

_____

_____

_____

_____

3. What are the serious side effects of steroid abuse in both men and women?

_____

_____

_____

_____

4. In what ways can untreated pain affect the elderly?

_____

_____

_____

_____

5. Why, during the Middle Ages, were tomatoes believed to be poisonous?

_____

_____

_____

_____

CHAPTER 1
ANSWER KEY

MULTIPLE CHOICE

1. b	6. d	11. b	16. c	21. a
2. c	7. b	12. a	17. c	22. c
3. a	8. a	13. d	18. d	23. a
4. a	9. b	14. c	19. b	24. c
5. d	10. c	15. d	20. b	25. b

MATCHING EXERCISES

Set 1	Set 2	Set 3
1. h	1. i	1. c
2. l	2. c	2. i
3. e	3. m	3. a
4. a	4. a	4. o
5. f	5. j	5. b
6. j	6. k	6. g
7. c	7. l	7. e
8. i	8. b	8. p
9. g	9. e	9. k
10. d	10. g	10. l

FILL IN THE BLANK

1. STAT
2. NPO
3. Negative Feedback
4. International System of Units/Metric
5. Angioplasty
6. Dermatology
7. Hepatitis
8. Cholecystectomy
9. Homeostasis
10. Etiology
11. Diagnosis
12. Prognosis
13. Microscopic
14. Hypothalamus
15. Vital

144

SHORT ANSWER

1. Signs and symptoms are terms often used interchangeably but each has its own specific definition. A sign is a more objective indicator (pulse rate) of illness, and a symptom is a more subjective (pain behind the eyes, for example) indicator of illness.

2. The two subdivisions of metabolism are anabolism and catabolism. Anabolism is the building up of complex structures using simpler compounds, like amino acids being used to build protein. Catabolism is the tearing down of complex material into smaller material, like the breaking down of food into its nutritional components.

3. *Anatomy* and *physiology* is the study of both the structure and function of the internal and external structure of plants, animals, or for the focus of this text, the human body.

4. The USCS system is based on the British Imperial System. USCS stands for United States Customary System and is used in the United States and Myanmar (formally Burma).

5. To maintain homeostasis when in a cold environment, the body begins to shiver, and the increased muscular activity generates heat. In addition, the body vasoconstricts the peripheral blood vessels, causing blood to be deeper from the skin surface where the heat would be lost to the cold environment.

CHAPTER 2
ANSWER KEY

MULTIPLE CHOICE

1. b	6. d	11. b	16. d	21. b
2. b	7. d	12. d	17. d	22. c
3. a	8. c	13. a	18. c	23. a
4. c	9. a	14. d	19. a	24. c
5. a	10. a	15. b	20. c	25. d

MATCHING EXERCISES

Set 1	Set 2	Set 3
1. h	1. e	1. f
2. j	2. l	2. d
3. g	3. h	3. b
4. a	4. a	4. c
5. i	5. g	5. g
6. e	6. c	6. j
7. f	7. j	7. a
8. l	8. i	8. i
9. c	9. b	9. e
10. b	10. f	10. k

FILL IN THE BLANK

1. dorsal
2. cheek
3. psoas
4. pleural
5. frontal/coronal
6. horizontal/transverse
7. pelvic
8. right lumbar
9. hypogastric
10. iliac
11. prone
12. epigastric
13. superior/proximal
14. medial
15. distal

SHORT ANSWER

1. The divisions of the abdominal regions include the right and left lower quadrants and the right and left upper quadrants.

2. The supine position would be advantageous if star watching, if on a respirator, if receiving an abdominal massage, if allowing for healing on the anterior surface of the body, if doing sit-ups, and if relieving lower back pain, to mention only a few.

3. From the patella, the calf muscles are posterior and distal or dorsal and inferior.

4. Proximal to the hips are the upper thigh or the femoral region. The leg or the crural region and the knee cap or the patella are inferior to the thigh on the anterior of the leg. The back of the knee or the popliteal region is posterior to the patella. The foot or the pedal region is the most distal part of the limb. The foot by itself includes the top or the dorsum and the sole or the plantar surface.

5. The coronal plane is a plane dividing the body or its parts into anterior and posterior sections or front and back sections.

LABELING ACTIVITY

See Figure 2–7 on page 31 in the textbook for comparison.

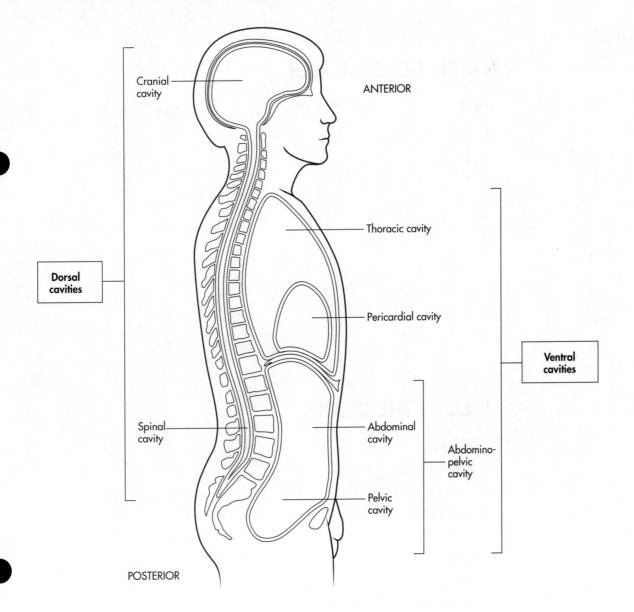

CHAPTER 3
ANSWER KEY

MULTIPLE CHOICE

1. b	6. a	11. b	16. c	21. a
2. d	7. c	12. c	17. a	22. c
3. d	8. b	13. a	18. b	23. a
4. c	9. d	14. b	19. a	24. c
5. a	10. c	15. b	20. b	25. b

MATCHING EXERCISES

Set 1	Set 2	Set 3
1. g	1. i	1. a
2. d	2. b	2. f
3. c	3. h	3. i
4. a	4. d	4. e
5. i	5. c	5. d
6. f	6. a	6. b
7. b	7. j	7. j
8. j	8. g	8. c
9. h	9. e	9. h
10. e	10. f	10. g

FILL IN THE BLANK

1. diffusion
2. phagocytosis
3. adenosine triphosphate
4. active transport pumps
5. DNA
6. benign
7. virus
8. vitamin K
9. spores
10. solute
11. phosphate
12. bacteria
13. mature RBC
14. cell
15. Malaria

SHORT ANSWER

1. The cell membrane is responsible for allowing materials in and out of the cell.

2. Protozoa can be found in water such as ponds and in soil.

3. Endoplasmic reticula (ER) are series of channels in the cytoplasm of the cell set up to serve as the road or transport system of the cell. The rough ER have ribosomes associated with their surface, and the smooth ER do not have ribosomes, and in addition to transport, they can produce steroids and lipids.

4. Passive transport requires no extra energy and includes such specific transports as diffusion, osmosis, and filtration. Active transport requires energy in the form of adenosine triphosphate and includes active pump, endocytosis, and exocytosis.

5. In filtration pressure is applied to force water and its dissolved material across a membrane.

LABELING ACTIVITY

See Figure 3–10 on page 56 in the textbook for comparison.

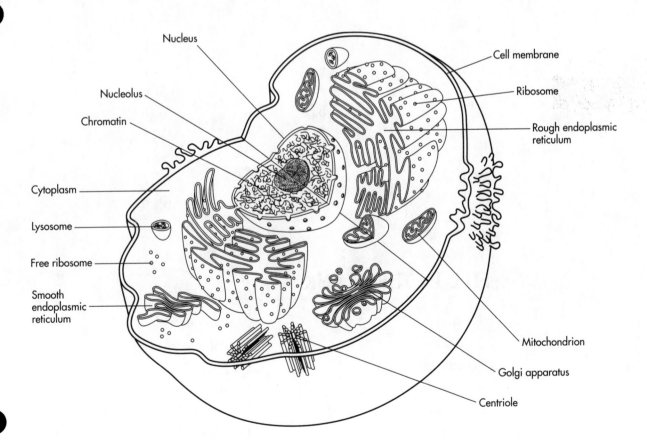

CHAPTER 4
ANSWER KEY

MULTIPLE CHOICE

1. c	6. c	11. a	16. d	21. a
2. b	7. b	12. a	17. c	22. d
3. a	8. b	13. c	18. b	23. d
4. c	9. a	14. a	19. a	24. c
5. a	10. b	15. d	20. b	25. d

MATCHING EXERCISES

Set 1	Set 2	Set 3
1. h	1. k	1. e
2. d	2. e	2. a
3. b	3. h	3. k
4. j	4. d	4. j
5. c	5. j	5. c
6. e	6. g	6. b
7. g	7. l	7. g
8. a	8. c	8. d
9. i	9. i	9. i
10. f	10. b	10. h

FILL IN THE BLANK

1. serous
2. heart
3. neuroglia
4. endocrine
5. digestive
6. circulatory
7. nervous and sensory
8. Vitamin D
9. axon
10. columnar
11. paired
12. striated
13. synovial
14. connective
15. lymphatic

SHORT ANSWER

1. The four types of tissue are epithelial, connective, muscle, and nervous. Epithelial tissue covers and lines much of the body and covers many parts found in the body. Connective tissue holds things together and provides structure and support. Muscle tissue contracts and by doing so moves bone and moves substances throughout and out of the body. Nervous tissue conducts impulses.

2. Cardiac muscle is found in the walls of the heart. Skeletal muscle is found attached to bone, and smooth muscle lines hollow organs and vessels. Both cardiac and smooth muscles are involuntary, and skeletal muscle is voluntary.

3. There are two types of nerve cells: the neuron conducts impulses and the neuroglia support and help hold neurons in place.

4. Serous membranes are composed of visceral and parietal layers, which reduce friction between different tissues and organs. The parietal layer lines cavities, and the visceral layer adheres to the organs.

5. Both the endocrine and nervous systems control the activity of virtually all the body organs. The nervous system does it by electrical impulses, and the endocrine system does it by chemicals called hormones.

LABELING ACTIVITY

See Figure 4–1 on page 71 in the textbook for comparison.

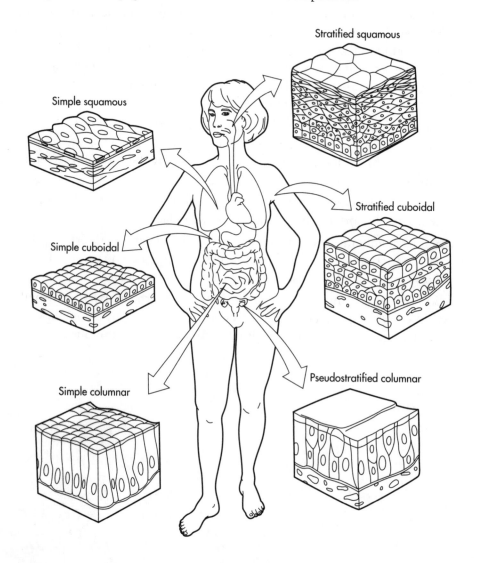

CHAPTER 5
ANSWER KEY

MULTIPLE CHOICE

1. c	6. c	11. a	16. a	21. c
2. c	7. b	12. d	17. a	22. c
3. a	8. a	13. c	18. c	23. a
4. c	9. c	14. b	19. a	24. c
5. e	10. b	15. d	20. b	25. a

MATCHING EXERCISES

Set 1	Set 2	Set 3
1. m	1. j	1. d
2. c	2. g	2. c
3. j	3. c	3. e
4. i	4. i	4. j
5. e	5. f	5. a
6. g	6. a	6. g
7. d	7. h	7. i
8. k	8. b	8. h
9. h	9. e	9. b
10. b	10. d	10. f

FILL IN THE BLANK

1. osteoporosis
2. congenital
3. cervical / lumbar
4. monocytes
5. plantar flexed
6. extension
7. mandible
8. body

9. vertebrocostal
10. hinge
11. ossification
12. arthritis
13. 206
14. comminuted
15. osteoclasts

SHORT ANSWER

1. The functions of the skeleton are to provide a framework, produce blood cells, protect organs, serve as a warehouse for mineral storage, and move with the assistance of the muscles.

2. The four types of bones are the flat, long, short, and irregular. Flat bones are platelike and include the sternum, ribs, and cranium. Long bones are longer than they are wide, and examples include bones of the arms and legs. Short bones are equal in width and length and found in the ankle and wrist. Irregular bones are odd-shaped bones like the hip and vertebrae.

3. The functions of the periosteum include covering the bone. The periosteum contains the blood vessels, nerves, and lymph that serve the bone itself. It also acts as an anchor for ligaments and tendons.

4. A ligament is a fibrous tissue connecting bone to bone usually over a joint. A tendon attaches muscle to bone.

5. Ribs 11 and 12 are called floating ribs because they are not attached anteriorly to anything—not to the sternum directly or indirectly as are the other 10 ribs.

LABELING ACTIVITY

See Figure 5–3 on page 101 in the textbook for comparison.

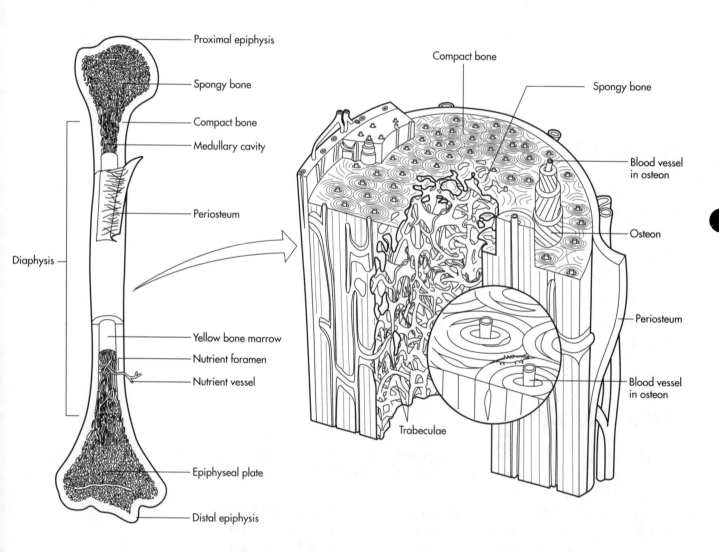

CHAPTER 6
ANSWER KEY

MULTIPLE CHOICE

1. a	6. d	11. c	16. c	21. c
2. b	7. a	12. c	17. c	22. b
3. b	8. a	13. d	18. a	23. c
4. a	9. c	14. a	19. c	24. d
5. c	10. b	15. d	20. d	25. d

MATCHING EXERCISES

Set 1	Set 2	Set 3
1. h	1. e	1. h
2. e	2. i	2. i
3. f	3. c	3. a
4. i	4. f	4. b
5. b	5. d	5. c
6. c	6. h	6. e
7. a	7. g	7. d
8. j	8. j	8. g
9. d	9. b	9. k
10. g	10. a	10. f

FILL IN THE BLANK

1. Intercalated disks
2. Peristalsis
3. Triceps
4. Flexion
5. Shivers
6. Glycogen
7. Sarcomere
8. Calcium
9. Acetylcholine
10. Z-lines
11. Quads
12. Synergist
13. Visceral
14. Heart
15. Ligament

SHORT ANSWER

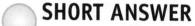

1. Due to their slower activity and lower metabolic rate, smooth muscles receive only moderate amounts of blood. They have difficulty repairing with moderate amounts of blood.

2. Functions of muscle include heat production and helping to maintain posture and stabilize joints.

3. Smooth muscles can be found surrounding blood vessels, the urinary bladder, the digestive tract, arrector pili in skin, and bronchi/bronchioles.

4. The functional contractile unit called the sarcomere has thick and thin filaments repeated several times through the muscle fiber and separated by a Z-line. These lines and filaments microscopically give muscle a striated or striped appearance.

5. Skeletal muscles are voluntary muscles that usually attach to bone. Smooth muscles are involuntary muscles found in organ walls, blood vessel walls, and airways. Cardiac muscle is involuntary and found as one of the layers surrounding the heart.

LABELING ACTIVITY

See Figure 4–8 on page 81 in the textbook for comparison.

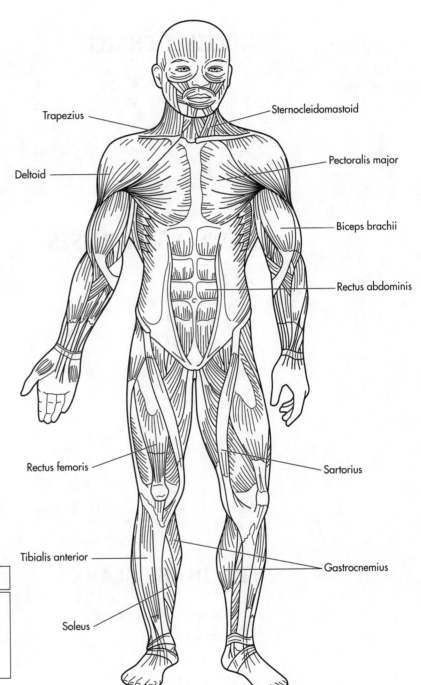

Trapezius

Sternocleidomastoid

Deltoid

Pectoralis major

Biceps brachii

Rectus abdominis

Rectus femoris

Sartorius

Tibialis anterior

Gastrocnemius

Soleus

Organ	Primary Functions
Skeletal muscles (700)	Provide skeletal movement, control openings of digestive tract, produce heat, support skeletal position, protect soft tissues

CHAPTER 7
ANSWER KEY

MULTIPLE CHOICE

1. d	6. c	11. a	16. d	21. c
2. c	7. b	12. b	17. b	22. a
3. c	8. c	13. a	18. a	23. c
4. a	9. a	14. d	19. a	24. a
5. d	10. a	15. d	20. c	25. b

MATCHING EXERCISES

Set 1	Set 2	Set 3
1. a	1. g	1. b
2. g	2. h	2. j
3. h	3. d	3. e
4. d	4. j	4. g
5. e	5. i	5. c
6. j	6. c	6. a
7. i	7. a	7. h
8. f	8. e	8. i
9. c	9. b	9. f
10. b	10. f	10. d

FILL IN THE BLANK

1. Collagenous and elastic
2. Melanoma
3. Herpes zoster
4. Arrector pili
5. Stratum corneum
6. Papule
7. 12
8. 3
9. Hematoma
10. Sebum
11. Third
12. 36
13. Root
14. Melanin
15. Bilirubin

SHORT ANSWER

1. Constriction of the arrector pili muscles shows up as goose flesh when we are chilled. When the hair stands up, pockets of nonmoving air are formed right above the skin, creating a dead air space that insulates the skin from the cooler surrounding environment.

2. Basal cell carcinoma usually spreads locally and can usually be successfully treated. Squamous cell carcinoma may develop deeper into tissue but rarely spreads to other tissue. Malignant melanoma develops deep in the skin and can spread throughout the body to various organs.

3. These sores are a result of a lack of blood flow to skin that has had pressure applied to a bony prominence.

4. Skin acts as storage for fatty tissue necessary for energy, keeps us from drying out, provides sensory impulse, regulates body temperature, and protects from disease-producing pathogens.

5. A pathologist, through hair analysis, can tell if an individual ingested certain drugs or other substances such as lead or arsenic.

LABELING ACTIVITY

See Figure 7–1 on page 151 in the textbook for comparison.

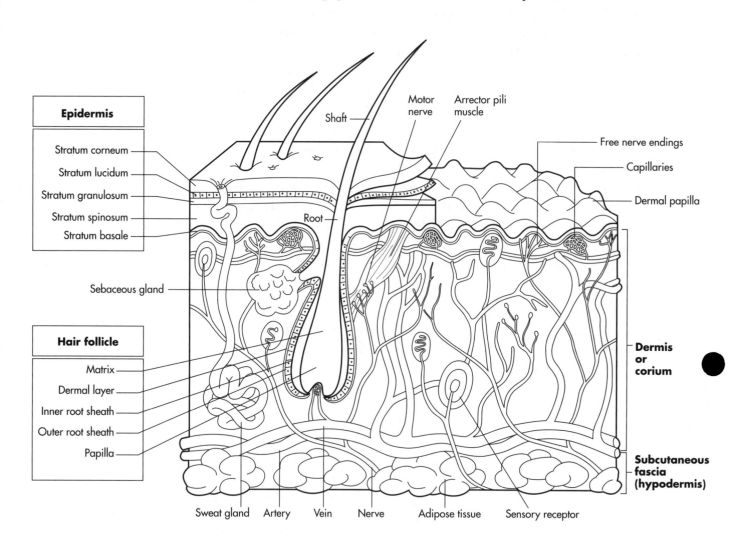

Epidermis
- Stratum corneum
- Stratum lucidum
- Stratum granulosum
- Stratum spinosum
- Stratum basale

Sebaceous gland

Hair follicle
- Matrix
- Dermal layer
- Inner root sheath
- Outer root sheath
- Papilla

Shaft

Motor nerve

Arrector pili muscle

Root

Free nerve endings

Capillaries

Dermal papilla

Dermis or corium

Subcutaneous fascia (hypodermis)

Sweat gland   Artery   Vein   Nerve   Adipose tissue   Sensory receptor

CHAPTER 8
ANSWER KEY

MULTIPLE CHOICE

1. b	6. a	11. a	16. c	21. c
2. b	7. c	12. a	17. a	22. a
3. c	8. c	13. c	18. b	23. c
4. b	9. d	14. b	19. a	24. c
5. d	10. d	15. a	20. b	25. c

MATCHING EXERCISES

Set 1	Set 2	Set 3
1. i	1. d	1. d
2. j	2. b	2. e
3. d	3. c	3. g
4. c	4. g	4. h
5. f	5. i	5. f
6. k	6. h	6. c
7. b	7. k	7. i
8. e	8. j	8. a
9. h	9. f	9. b
10. g	10. e	10. j

FILL IN THE BLANK

1. resting and digesting
2. synapse
3. neurotransmitter
4. ventral/dorsal/lateral
5. epidural/dura mater
6. anterior median fissure/posterior median sulcus
7. conus medullaris
8. dorsal/ventral
9. reflex
10. median
11. startle/withdrawal/vestibular
12. meninges
13. excited
14. sodium
15. multiple sclerosis

SHORT ANSWER

1. The spinal cord ends at lumbar-2 in a pointed structure called the conus medullaris. Hanging from the conus medullaris is a bunch of paired spinal nerves (L2-coccygeal), dangling loosely. This is the cauda equina, which looks like its name, "horse's tail."

2. When the doctor taps on your knee, the hammer gently stretches the tendon associated with the quadriceps muscle, which in turn stretches the muscle itself. The sensory neurons in the quadriceps muscle pick up on this stretch and send their impulses to the spinal cord. The sensory neurons then synapse with the motor neurons in the spinal cord, and the motor neurons send impulses back down to the quads. As a protective mechanism, the motor neurons signal the quadriceps to contract, or shorten. This shortening pulls on the insertion, which is the leg, and the leg extends at the knee.

3. In local potential, the size of the stimulus determines the excitement of the cell. A big stimulus causes a bigger depolarization than a small stimulus.

4. The peripheral nervous system includes the nerves outside of the brain and spinal cord, meaning it includes the cranial and spinal nerves.

5. Action potential is all-or-none; once it starts, it will always finish and will always be the same size, whereas the local potential varies in size.

LABELING ACTIVITY

See Figure 4–10 on page 83 in the textbook for comparison.

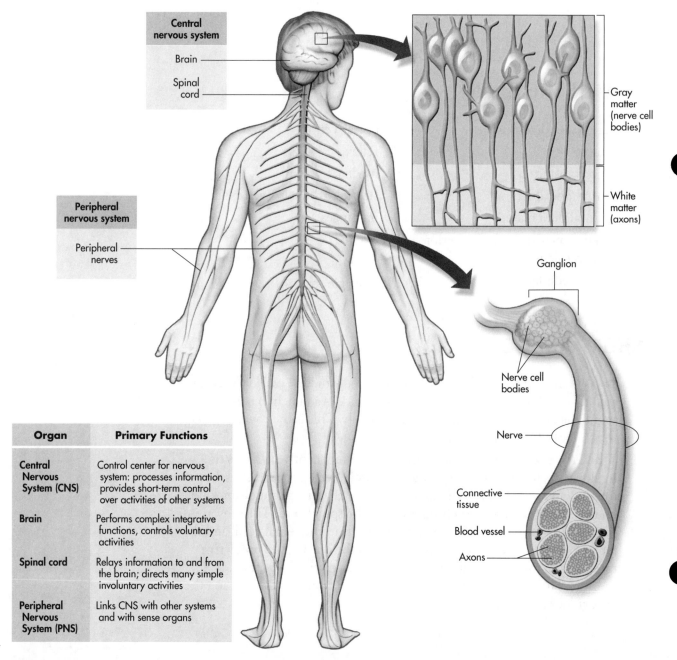

Organ	Primary Functions
Central Nervous System (CNS)	Control center for nervous system: processes information, provides short-term control over activities of other systems
Brain	Performs complex integrative functions, controls voluntary activities
Spinal cord	Relays information to and from the brain; directs many simple involuntary activities
Peripheral Nervous System (PNS)	Links CNS with other systems and with sense organs

CHAPTER 9
ANSWER KEY

MULTIPLE CHOICE

1. a	6. d	11. b	16. b	21. d
2. a	7. c	12. c	17. b	22. c
3. c	8. a	13. b	18. a	23. a
4. b	9. b	14. d	19. d	24. c
5. d	10. b	15. b	20. a	25. a

MATCHING EXERCISES

Set 1	Set 2	Set 3
1. e	1. i	1. d
2. k	2. l	2. i
3. h	3. j	3. f
4. l	4. k	4. h
5. j	5. d	5. e
6. a	6. g	6. b
7. d	7. b	7. a
8. i	8. c	8. g
9. c	9. h	9. c
10. b	10. f	10. j

FILL IN THE BLANK

1. Cerebrum/brain stem/cerebellum
2. Longitudinal
3. Gyri
4. Vagus/Glossopharyngeal
5. Vision
6. Lateral fissure
7. Midbrain/pons/medulla oblongata
8. Cortex
9. Temporal lobe
10. Cerebral spinal fluid
11. Spinocerebellar
12. Adrenal
13. Recticular
14. Sympathetic
15. Motor

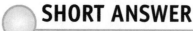

SHORT ANSWER

1. The left side of the body is controlled by the right side of the cerebral cortex, and the right side of the body is controlled by the left brain.

2. The dura mater, the most superficial of the brain's meninges, is fused to the inside of the skull.

3. The purpose of convolutions is to increase the surface area of the brain so more brain can be packed into a smaller space.

4. All 31 pairs of spinal nerves are mixed (motor and sensory). There are only 12 pairs of cranial nerves and not all are mixed. Some are mostly motor, such as the trochlear nerve, and some are mostly sensory, such as the olfactory nerve.

5. Both the sympathetic and parasympathetic nervous systems have limited effects on the skeletal muscle. The autonomic nervous system controls involuntary muscles. The sympathetic nervous system increases heart rate and increases blood pressure by constricting blood vessels. The parasympathetic nervous system decreases heart rate, decreases blood pressure, and increases digestive activity.

LABELING ACTIVITY

See Figure 9–3 on page 202 in the textbook for comparison.

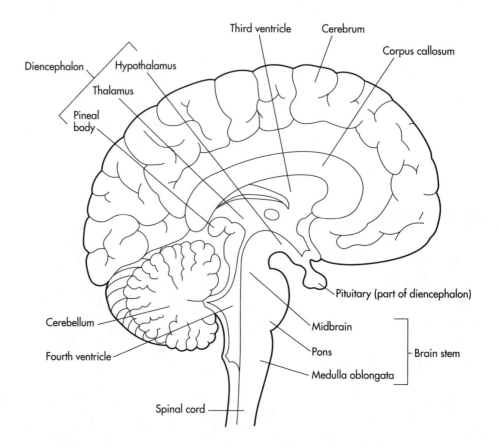

CHAPTER 10
ANSWER KEY

MULTIPLE CHOICE

1. d	6. d	11. a	16. d	21. d
2. c	7. a	12. d	17. a	22. c
3. a	8. c	13. a	18. d	23. b
4. b	9. b	14. b	19. b	24. c
5. d	10. b	15. a	20. a	25. b

MATCHING EXERCISES

Set 1	Set 2	Set 3
1. f	1. f	1. b
2. c	2. b	2. i
3. i	3. k	3. c
4. d	4. g	4. g
5. g	5. i	5. h
6. h	6. c	6. a
7. e	7. d	7. j
8. j	8. j	8. d
9. a	9. h	9. f
10. b	10. a	10. e

FILL IN THE BLANK

1. Oxytocin
2. Adenohypophysis
3. Thymus Gland
4. Insulin/Glucagon
5. Addison's Disease
6. Thyroid-Stimulating Hormone (TSH)
7. Prolactin/Oxytocin
8. Pituitary
9. Skin
10. Antidiuretic Hormone
11. Humoral/Hormonal/Neural
12. Adrenal cortex
13. Parathyroid
14. Hormones
15. Progesterone

SHORT ANSWER

1. Endocrine glands secrete chemical messengers called hormones into the bloodstream, whereas exocrine glands secrete their substances into ducts that lead to either a lumen or to the outside of the body, such as digestive enzymes from the pancreas or sweat from the sweat glands (sudoriferous glands).

2. Mutual side effects of steroid abuse in both men and women include aggression, cardiovascular diseases, and increased cholesterol.

3. Alcohol and caffeinated coffee both suppress a hormone called antidiuretic hormone (ADH). ADH is responsible for water uptake or water reabsorption in the kidney. If suppressed, it allows excessive water to be excreted rather than reabsorbed.

4. Humoral pertains to body fluids or substances. Humoral control is hormone level control of the internal environment by monitoring body fluids.

5. Steroid hormones can bind to sites inside the cells. They are lipid molecules that can pass easily through the target cell's membrane. These hormones then can interact directly with the cell's DNA to change cell activity.

LABELING ACTIVITY

See Figure 4–11 on page 84 in the textbook for comparison.

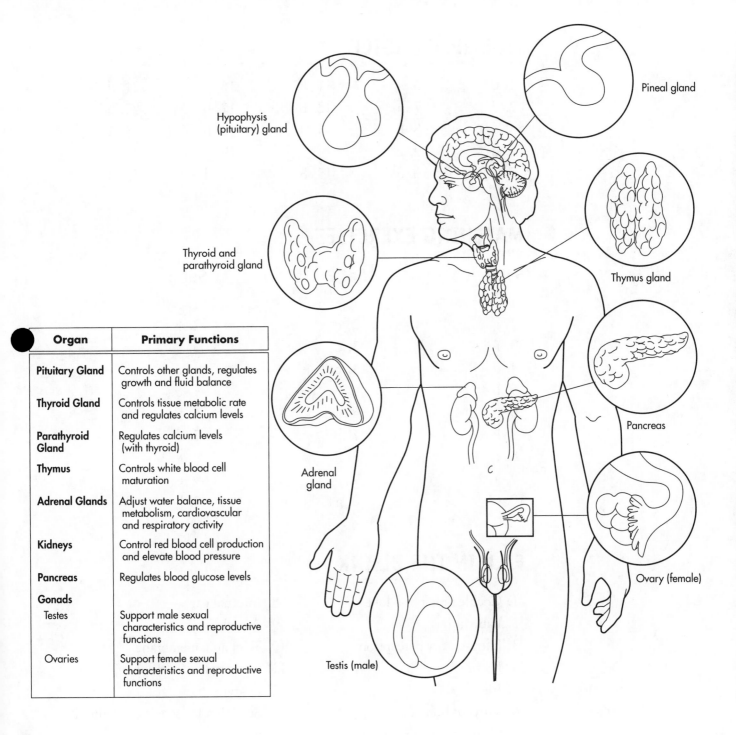

Organ	Primary Functions
Pituitary Gland	Controls other glands, regulates growth and fluid balance
Thyroid Gland	Controls tissue metabolic rate and regulates calcium levels
Parathyroid Gland	Regulates calcium levels (with thyroid)
Thymus	Controls white blood cell maturation
Adrenal Glands	Adjust water balance, tissue metabolism, cardiovascular and respiratory activity
Kidneys	Control red blood cell production and elevate blood pressure
Pancreas	Regulates blood glucose levels
Gonads	
Testes	Support male sexual characteristics and reproductive functions
Ovaries	Support female sexual characteristics and reproductive functions

CHAPTER 11
ANSWER KEY

MULTIPLE CHOICE

1. d	6. a	11. b	16. c	21. d
2. d	7. a	12. b	17. b	22. b
3. c	8. b	13. d	18. b	23. a
4. d	9. b	14. a	19. a	24. c
5. a	10. d	15. b	20. d	25. d

MATCHING EXERCISES

Set 1	Set 2	Set 3
1. j	1. e	1. g
2. g	2. d	2. k
3. f	3. c	3. j
4. d	4. b	4. i
5. b	5. i	5. c
6. i	6. a	6. h
7. k	7. h	7. a
8. e	8. k	8. f
9. a	9. j	9. e
10. c	10. g	10. b

FILL IN THE BLANK

1. Cochlea/temporal lobe
2. Labyrinth
3. Extrasensory perception
4. Lacrimal
5. Iris
6. Vitreous humor
7. Ceruminous/lubricate and protect ear
8. Internal ear
9. Auricle
10. Tympanic membrane
11. Perilymph and endolymph
12. Pharynx
13. Semicircular canals/cerebellum
14. Pink eye
15. Special

SHORT ANSWER

1. The eyelids close over the eye much like the lens cover of a camera to protect it from intense light, foreign particles, or impact injuries. The eyelids also contain sebaceous glands, which secrete the oily substance sebum onto the eyelid to keep it soft, pliable, and a little sticky to trap particles.

2. During adaptation there is continued sensory stimulation causing the sensors to desensitize or adapt. An example is when the temperature has not changed yet the body no longer feels the extreme hot or cold. It seems to be getting more neutral.

3. Accommodation combines changes in the size of the pupil and the lens curvature to make sure the image converges in the same place on the retina and therefore is properly focused.

4. The three layers of the eye are the sclera, the outermost layer commonly called the "white" of the eye; the middle layer, called the choroid, which contains the iris and pupil; and the deepest layer, called the retina, containing the nerve endings that receive and interpret the rays of light into what we see.

5. The three types of auditory conduction are sound, bone, and sensorineural conductions. Sound conduction is the vibration of the tympanic membrane by the actual sound waves. Bone conduction is the amplification of the waves by the ossicles or ear bones. The last is the sensorineural conduction, the process by which the cochlear fluid vibrates the hairs to send nerve impulses to the temporal lobe of the brain where they are interpreted as sound.

LABELING ACTIVITY

See Figure 11–3 on page 254 in the textbook for comparison.

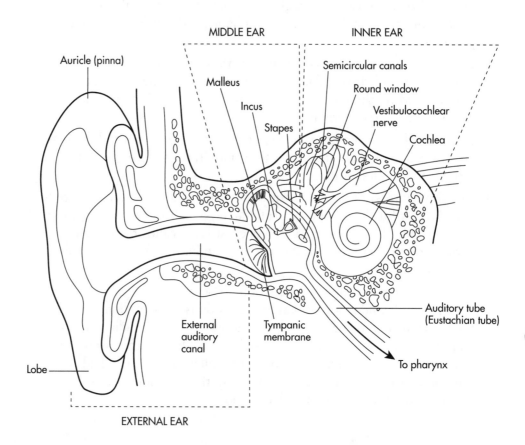

MIDDLE EAR   INNER EAR

Auricle (pinna)

Malleus

Incus

Stapes

Semicircular canals

Round window

Vestibulocochlear nerve

Cochlea

External auditory canal

Tympanic membrane

Auditory tube (Eustachian tube)

To pharynx

Lobe

EXTERNAL EAR

CHAPTER 12
ANSWER KEY

 MULTIPLE CHOICE

1. b	6. b	11. c	16. a	21. a
2. b	7. c	12. c	17. b	22. c
3. d	8. c	13. a	18. c	23. b
4. d	9. a	14. c	19. c	24. d
5. b	10. b	15. a	20. d	25. a

MATCHING EXERCISES

Set 1	Set 2	Set 3
1. i	1. d	1. f
2. f	2. c	2. j
3. h	3. f	3. a
4. d	4. i	4. g
5. g	5. j	5. h
6. a	6. h	6. i
7. b	7. e	7. b
8. c	8. a	8. e
9. j	9. g	9. d
10. e	10. b	10. c

FILL IN THE BLANK

1. Away from
2. Interventricular septum
3. QRS
4. Gases/nutrients/wastes/hormones
5. Formed elements/plasma
6. Liver/K
7. Interatrial septum
8. tricuspid or right AV
9. increase
10. right atrium
11. calcium
12. fibrin
13. cholesterol
14. sphygmomanometer/stethoscope
15. Inferior vena cava/superior vena cava

SHORT ANSWER

1. Agglutination is when the surface antigens on the red blood cells stick (clump) together. This is a potentially dangerous situation. Coagulation is clotting, usually at a site of injury, and it uses clotting proteins dissolved in the plasma as well as vitamin K. Clotting prevents blood loss when a vessel is compromised.

2. The vessel that leaves the right ventricle is called the pulmonary trunk, which leads to the pulmonary arteries. The arteries and the trunk itself route deoxygenated blood toward the lungs. Since it carries blood away from the heart, the vessels are termed arteries. The pulmonary veins, on the other hand, route blood from the lungs back to the heart. The blood is oxygen-rich. Since it approaches or leads to the heart, these vessels are termed veins. Fetal circulation follows the same principle.

3. Many substances are carried by the blood. Besides water, there are CO_2, a little oxygen, electrolytes like sodium, potassium and chloride,

nutrients, hormones, plasma proteins like albumin, fibrinogen and globulin.

4. The sympathetic nervous system increases heart rate and force of contraction. The parasympathetic division of the autonomic nervous system decreases both the pulse (rate) and the force of contraction.

5. The walls of the heart receive blood supply from the coronary arteries (right and left) that branch directly off the ascending aorta. The right coronary artery provides blood for the right ventricle, posterior portion of the interventricular septum, and inferior parts of the heart. The left coronary artery provides blood to the left lateral and anterior walls of the left ventricle and portions of the right ventricle and interventricular septum.

 # LABELING ACTIVITY

This illustration should be color-coded per Figure 12–1 on page 271 in the text.

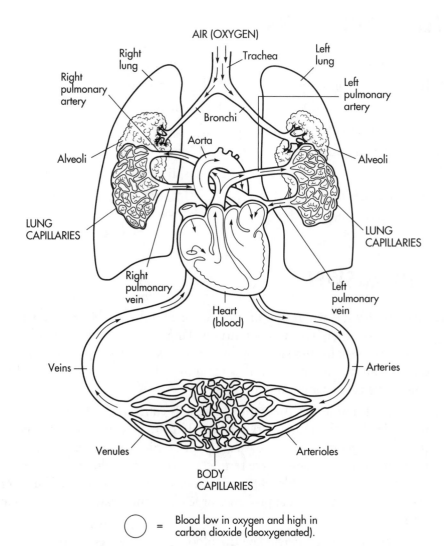

CHAPTER 13
ANSWER KEY

MULTIPLE CHOICE

1. d	6. b	11. b	16. a	21. b
2. b	7. a	12. d	17. b	22. a
3. a	8. b	13. b	18. c	23. a
4. c	9. a	14. c	19. b	24. d
5. a	10. d	15. a	20. d	25. d

MATCHING EXERCISES

Set 1	Set 2	Set 3
1. g	1. h	1. e
2. i	2. e	2. d
3. c	3. b	3. j
4. k	4. j	4. k
5. f	5. i	5. i
6. h	6. d	6. b
7. b	7. f	7. h
8. d	8. a	8. g
9. e	9. c	9. a
10. j	10. g	10. f

FILL IN THE BLANK

1. 80 percent
2. nasopharynx/oropharynx/ laryngopharynx
3. larynx
4. windpipe
5. 450,000
6. hilum
7. diaphragm
8. 3, 2
9. alveoli
10. 12, 7, 2
11. apex
12. decreases
13. alveoler-capillary membrane
14. increases/increases
15. middle ear/pharynx

SHORT ANSWER

1. Nose hairs play an important role as a gross-particle filter.

2. The primary functions of the respiratory system include bringing oxygen from the atmosphere into the bloodstream and removing carbon dioxide from the bloodstream.

3. Other muscles of inspiration include the external intercostals, sternocleidomastoid, scalenes, pectoralis major, and pectoralis minor that all pull the rib cage up, increasing the volume and decreasing the pressure. Inspiration then occurs.

4. Internal respiration is transport of oxygenated blood to the body via the cardiovascular system to the cells and tissue where gas exchange takes place: oxygen moves into the cells and carbon dioxide leaves the cells, moving into the blood capillaries. External respiration is the exchange of gases in the lungs where oxygen is moved from lung alveoli into the pulmonary capillaries, and carbon dioxide moves from the pulmonary capillaries into the lung alveoli.

5. The right main stem of the primary bronchus branches off at a 20- to 30-degree angle from the midline and the left branches off at a 40- to 60-degree angle. The lesser angle of the right makes it easier for foreign bodies that are accidentally breathed in to lodge in that lung.

LABELING ACTIVITY

See Figure 13–1 on page 305 in the textbook for comparison.

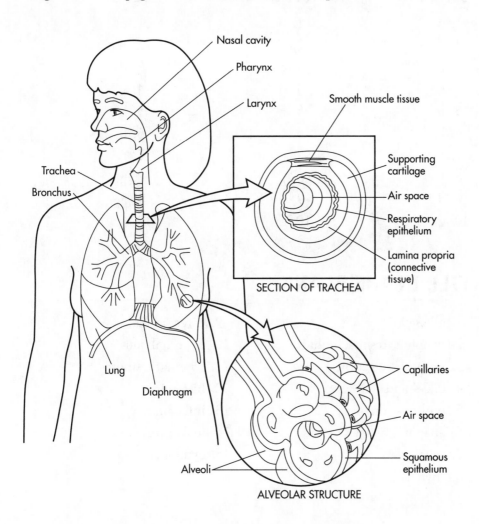

Nasal cavity

Pharynx

Larynx

Smooth muscle tissue

Supporting cartilage

Air space

Respiratory epithelium

Lamina propria (connective tissue)

SECTION OF TRACHEA

Trachea

Bronchus

Lung

Diaphragm

Capillaries

Air space

Squamous epithelium

Alveoli

ALVEOLAR STRUCTURE

CHAPTER 14
ANSWER KEY

MULTIPLE CHOICE

1. a	6. d	11. c	16. b	21. d
2. d	7. c	12. b	17. b	22. b
3. a	8. a	13. b	18. a	23. d
4. a	9. a	14. b	19. c	24. b
5. d	10. d	15. d	20. a	25. d

MATCHING EXERCISES

Set 1	Set 2	Set 3
1. c	1. b	1. c
2. a	2. a	2. h
3. e	3. c	3. d
4. f	4. d	4. i
5. b	5. h	5. b
6. h	6. i	6. e
7. j	7. g	7. f
8. i	8. j	8. g
9. d	9. f	9. a
10. g	10. e	10. j

FILL IN THE BLANK

1. allergy
2. lymphocytes/macrophages
3. negative selection
4. CD-4 and CD-8
5. proliferation
6. anaphylaxis/low
7. subclavian
8. thymus
9. three
10. hypothalamus
11. lymphatic sinuses
12. histamine
13. inflammatory
14. leukocytes
15. cytokines

SHORT ANSWER

1. Immune deficiency can be caused by genetics, chemicals, radiation exposure, or even medication. Immune-compromised clients include those with severe combined immune deficiency, a genetic disorder, leukemia, some forms of anemia, and patients undergoing chemotherapy or taking immune-suppressing drugs after organ transplant.

2. Lymph nodes filter lymph fluid and destroy pathogens with the WBCs that are housed in the nodes.

3. The spleen is structurally similar to lymph nodes, but instead of having lymphatic sinuses, the spleen has blood sinuses.

4. A fever is a deliberate attempt by the immune system to destroy the pathogens that invade the body.

5. CD-4 cells are necessary for the proliferation of B cells and cytotoxic T cells.

LABELING ACTIVITY

See Figure 4–14 on page 87 in the textbook for comparison.

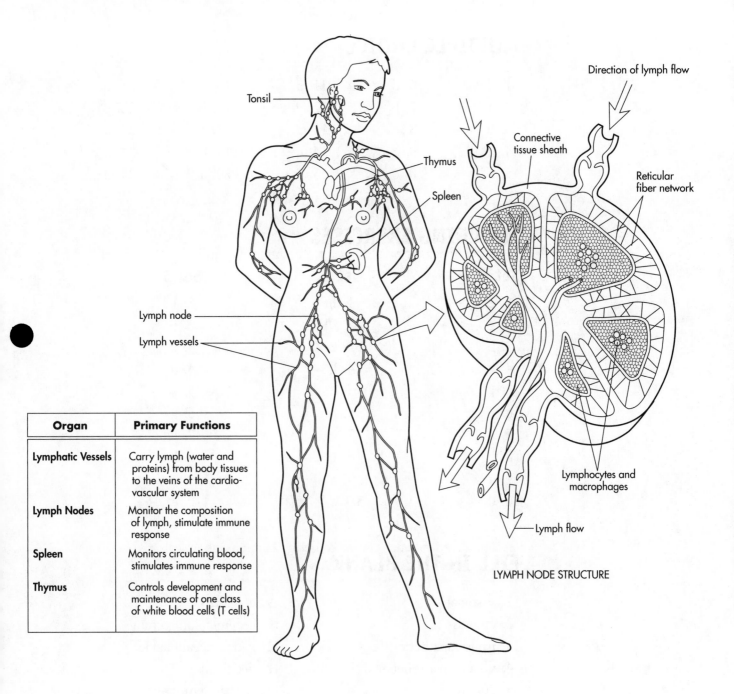

Organ	Primary Functions
Lymphatic Vessels	Carry lymph (water and proteins) from body tissues to the veins of the cardio-vascular system
Lymph Nodes	Monitor the composition of lymph, stimulate immune response
Spleen	Monitors circulating blood, stimulates immune response
Thymus	Controls development and maintenance of one class of white blood cells (T cells)

LYMPH NODE STRUCTURE

CHAPTER 15
ANSWER KEY

MULTIPLE CHOICE

1. d	6. d	11. a	16. d	21. d
2. a	7. b	12. d	17. b	22. c
3. b	8. c	13. a	18. a	23. a
4. a	9. d	14. c	19. c	24. a
5. a	10. c	15. a	20. a	25. d

MATCHING EXERCISES

Set 1	Set 2	Set 3
1. c	1. l/f	1. l
2. g	2. f/l	2. b
3. h	3. a	3. i
4. k	4. k	4. d
5. j	5. b	5. j
6. f	6. j/h	6. g
7. i	7. e	7. k
8. b	8. i	8. h
9. a	9. g	9. c
10. d	10. c	10. e

FILL IN THE BLANK

1. vestigial
2. cuspids
3. parasympathetic
4. visceral peritoneum
5. 20
6. defecation
7. alimentary
8. diarrhea
9. epiglottis
10. cecum/colon/rectum
11. pancreas/gallbladder
12. deciduous
13. cardiac sphincter
14. amylase
15. constipation

SHORT ANSWER

1. Villi, plicae circularis, and microvilli provide an incredible increase in the surface area of the small intestine, which increases the effectiveness of the absorption of nutrients.

2. Lactose in milk products is not sufficiently digested. Normal bacteria found in the intestine utilize those undigested sugars with gas production as a by-product.

3. Mucous cells generate a thick layer of mucus that shields the stomach lining from the effect of HCl.

4. Parotid glands are located slightly inferior and anterior to the ears. Submandibular glands are on both sides along the inner surface of the mandible or lower jaw. Sublingual glands are under the tongue.

5. Digestion is necessary so nutrients can be absorbed by the lining of the digestive tract.

LABELING ACTIVITY

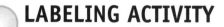

See Figure 4–15 on page 88 in the textbook for comparison.

Organ	Primary Functions
Salivary Glands	Provide lubrication, produce buffers and the enzymes that begin digestion
Pharynx	Passageway connected to esophagus
Esophagus	Delivers food to stomach
Stomach	Secretes acids and enzymes
Small Intestine	Secretes digestive enzymes, absorbs nutrients
Liver	Secretes bile, regulates blood chemistry
Gallbladder	Stores bile for release into small intestine
Pancreas	Secretes digestive enzymes and buffers; contains endocrine cells
Large Intestine	Removes water from fecal material, stores waste

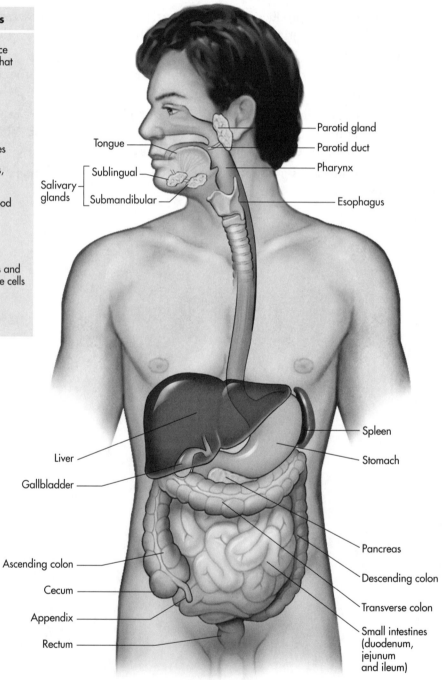

Tongue

Salivary glands — Sublingual
              — Submandibular

Parotid gland
Parotid duct
Pharynx
Esophagus

Liver
Gallbladder

Spleen
Stomach

Ascending colon
Cecum
Appendix
Rectum

Pancreas
Descending colon
Transverse colon
Small intestines (duodenum, jejunum and ileum)

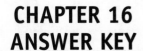

CHAPTER 16
ANSWER KEY

MULTIPLE CHOICE

1. a	6. c	11. b	16. d	21. d
2. d	7. b	12. c	17. b	22. b
3. b	8. a	13. b	18. a	23. c
4. a	9. c	14. c	19. c	24. a
5. b	10. b	15. d	20. c	25. b

MATCHING EXERCISES

Set 1	Set 2	Set 3
1. b	1. e	1. d
2. f	2. c	2. e
3. i	3. h	3. a
4. g	4. d	4. j
5. a	5. i	5. b
6. e	6. j	6. g
7. h	7. f	7. c
8. j	8. g	8. i
9. c	9. b	9. h
10. d	10. a	10. f

FILL IN THE BLANK

1. filtration/secretion/reabsorption
2. afferent arterioles/efferent arterioles
3. renal corpuscle/renal tubule
4. caffeinated coffee/alcohol
5. lithotripsy
6. diabetic nephropathy
7. aldosterone
8. diabetes mellitus
9. renal vein/ureter/renal artery
10. renal pelvis
11. nephron
12. descending loop
13. secretion
14. efferent arterioles and peritubular capillaries
15. parasympathetic

SHORT ANSWER

1. Urinary tract infections are more common in women than men because a woman's urethra is shorter than a man's and fecal matter can more easily travel to the urinary bladder and up the urinary tract.

2. As systemic blood pressure increases over normal range of BP, the afferent arterioles leading into the glomerulus constrict, decreasing the amount of blood getting into the glomerulus. Autoregulation protects the delicate filters from repeated rapid changes in blood pressure.

3. If there is too much acid in the blood, hydrogen ions, which cause acidity and the pH to drop, will be excreted to a greater level in the urine. At the same time, more bicarbonate ions will be reabsorbed back into the acidic blood, pulling the pH up to a more neutral level.

4. Aldosterone increases the reabsorption of sodium. In contrast, atrial natriuretic hormone (peptide) decreases sodium reabsorption.

5. With massive blood loss, blood pressure falls. To maintain normal blood pressure, there is widespread vasoconstriction. The afferent arterioles of the kidneys get smaller, greatly decreasing blood supply to the nephrons. Tissues soon become ischemic and begin to die.

LABELING ACTIVITY

See Figure 4–16 on page 89 in the textbook for comparison.

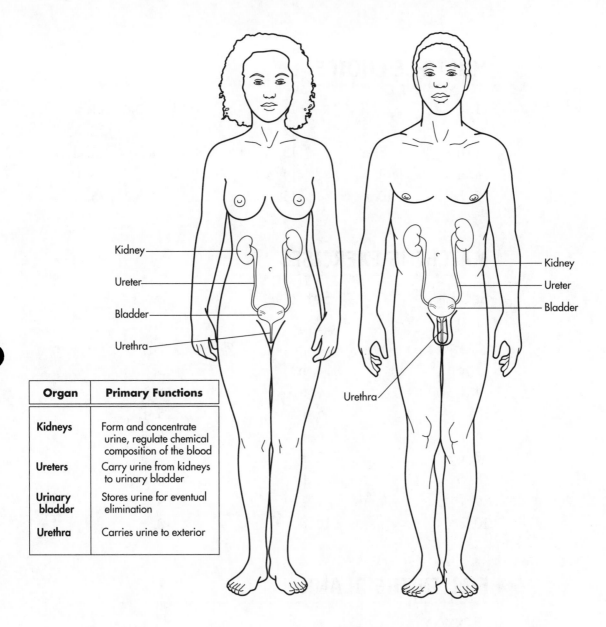

Organ	Primary Functions
Kidneys	Form and concentrate urine, regulate chemical composition of the blood
Ureters	Carry urine from kidneys to urinary bladder
Urinary bladder	Stores urine for eventual elimination
Urethra	Carries urine to exterior

CHAPTER 17
ANSWER KEY

MULTIPLE CHOICE

1. c	6. b	11. d	16. b	21. a
2. c	7. c	12. c	17. a	22. a
3. d	8. a	13. b	18. d	23. d
4. a	9. a	14. a	19. c	24. b
5. b	10. c	15. d	20. c	25. a

MATCHING EXERCISES

Set 1	Set 2	Set 3
1. d	1. c	1. d
2. j	2. g	2. j
3. e	3. h	3. e
4. f	4. a	4. f
5. b	5. i	5. b
6. a	6. j	6. a
7. g	7. f	7. g
8. h	8. b	8. h
9. i	9. e	9. i
10. c	10. d	10. c

FILL IN THE BLANK

1. XX/XY
2. semen/urine
3. spermatogenesis
4. erection
5. alveoli
6. pudendal
7. luteal
8. seminal vesicles
9. 46
10. pituitary gland
11. foreskin
12. fundus
13. testes
14. before birth
15. cervix

SHORT ANSWER

1. The first menstrual period is called the menarche, and menopause represents the ending of menstrual activity.

2. The three stages of labor are the dilation, delivery, and placental stages. The dilation stage is when contraction of the uterine smooth muscle is noted and the cervix also dilates to allow passage of the fetus's head. The delivery stage is noted with the presenting of the fetus's head, called crowning. The mouth is suctioned at this stage. The placental stage is when the placenta or afterbirth is delivered with the final uterine contraction.

3. Estrogen stimulates the proliferation of the uterine lining, and progesterone maintains the buildup of the endometrium.

4. The 23rd pair of chromosomes is the sex chromosomes. These are called sex chromosomes because their identity determines the sex of a baby. XX is female and XY is male. The female always contributes an X, but the male can contribute either an X or Y chromosome. The male actually determines the sex of the baby by contributing either an X chromosome for a girl or a Y chromosome for a boy.

5. Sperm is propelled from the epididymis of the scrotal sac into the vas deferens, which then carries the sperm into the pelvic cavity. As the sperm passes the seminal vesicles, sugar and chemicals are added to sperm, and then the substance enters the ejaculatory duct. As the ejaculatory duct passes through the prostate gland, prostatic fluid is added, liquefying the semen. The semen passes by the bulbourethral glands, which add mucus to the semen. The semen is then released into the vagina.

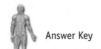

LABELING ACTIVITY

See Figure 4–17 on page 90 in the textbook for comparison.

Organ	Primary Functions (female)
Ovaries	Produce ova (eggs) and hormones
Uterine Tubes	Deliver ova or embryo to uterus; normal site of fertilization
Uterus	Site of development of offspring
Vagina	Site of sperm deposition; birth canal at delivery; provides passage of fluids during menstruation
External Genitalia	
Clitoris	Erectile organ, produces pleasurable sensations during sexual act
Labia	Contain glands that lubricate entrance to vagina
Mammary Glands	Produce milk that nourishes newborn infant

Organ	Primary Functions (male)
Testes	Produce sperm and hormones
Accessory Organs	
Epididymis	Site of sperm maturation
Ductus deferens (sperm duct)	Conducts sperm between epididymis and prostate
Seminal vesicles	Secrete fluid that makes up much of the volume of semen
Prostate	Secretes buffers and fluid
Urethra	Conducts semen to exterior
External Genitalia	
Penis	Erectile organ used to deposit sperm in the vagina of a female; produces pleasurable sensations during sexual act
Scrotum	Surrounds and positions the testes

Mammary glands

Fallopian tubes

Ovary

Uterus

Vagina

Prostate

Testis

Vas deferens

Urethra

Penis

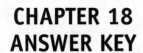

CHAPTER 18
ANSWER KEY

MULTIPLE CHOICE

1. a	6. b	11. d	16. d	21. b
2. a	7. c	12. d	17. b	22. b
3. a	8. c	13. d	18. a	23. d
4. d	9. b	14. c	19. d	24. b
5. a	10. b	15. d	20. c	25. c

MATCHING EXERCISES

Set 1	Set 2	Set 3
1. c	1. g	1. j
2. d	2. a	2. d
3. g	3. h	3. f
4. h	4. b	4. g
5. j	5. i	5. b
6. b	6. c	6. e
7. e	7. j	7. i
8. i	8. d	8. h
9. a	9. e	9. c
10. f	10. f	10. a

FILL IN THE BLANK

1. Egyptians
2. Jamestown, Virginia
3. Polypharmacy
4. 50
5. 35
6. Muscle mass/bone density/fat
7. Cervix
8. Testosterone
9. breast
10. 450,000
11. Radiation
12. Sentinel lymph node mapping and biopsy
13. Emphysema/Bronchitis/Asthma
14. Congenital Insensitivity to Pain and Anhidrosis
15. Hair

SHORT ANSWER

1. Cauliflower-like growths on the penis and vagina.

2. Minimize time in the sun between 10 a.m. and 4 p.m.; wear long-sleeved shirts, brimmed hat, sunglasses, sunscreen.

3. Kidney damage, liver damage, increased risk of heart disease, irritability, and aggressive behavior.

4. Changes in personality, such as becoming agitated, quiet, withdrawn, sad, confused, depressed, or grumpy, and behavior such as crying, swearing, grunting, loss of appetite, and wincing.

5. The acidic tomatoes served on pewter plates leached out the lead, which was consumed and led to lead poisoning.